ARCHAEA - NEW BIOCATALYSTS, NOVEL PHARMACEUTICALS AND VARIOUS BIOTECHNOLOGICAL APPLICATIONS

Edited by **Haïtham Sghaier, Afef Najjari**
and **Kais Ghedira**

Archaea - New Biocatalysts, Novel Pharmaceuticals and Various Biotechnological Applications
http://dx.doi.org/10.5772/65163
Edited by Haïtham Sghaier, Afef Najjari and Kais Ghedira

Contributors

Rosa María Martínez-Espinosa, Javier Torregrosa-Crespo, Carmen Pire, Jean-François Brugere, Wajdi Ben Hania, Nathalie Ballet, Pascal Vandekerckove, Paul W. O'Toole, Bernard Ollivier, Victoria Guixé, Victor Castro-Fernandez, Ricardo A Zamora, Alejandra Herrera-Morande, Gabriel Vallejos, Felipe Gonzalez-Ordenes, Hirokazu Suzuki, Tatsuki Mizuno, Takashi Ohshiro, Haitham Sghaier

Published by InTech

Janeza Trdine 9, 51000 Rijeka, Croatia

Notice

Statements and opinions expressed in the chapters are these of the individual contributors and not necessarily those of the editors or publisher. No responsibility is accepted for the accuracy of information contained in the published chapters. The publisher assumes no responsibility for any damage or injury to persons or property arising out of the use of any materials, instructions, methods or ideas contained in the book.

Publishing Process Manager Romina Rovan
Technical Editor SPi Global
Cover InTech Design team

First published October, 2017
Printed in Croatia
Legal deposit, Croatia: National and University Library in Zagreb

Additional hard copies can be obtained from orders@intechopen.com

Archaea - New Biocatalysts, Novel Pharmaceuticals and Various Biotechnological Applications, Edited by Haïtham Sghaier, Afef Najjari and Kais Ghedira
p. cm.
Print ISBN 978-953-51-3569-2
Online ISBN 978-953-51-3570-8

For EU product safety concerns:
IN TECH d.o.o., Prolaz Marije Krucifikse Kozulić 3, 51000 Rijeka, Croatia,
info@intechopen.com or visit our website at intechopen.com.

Meet the editors

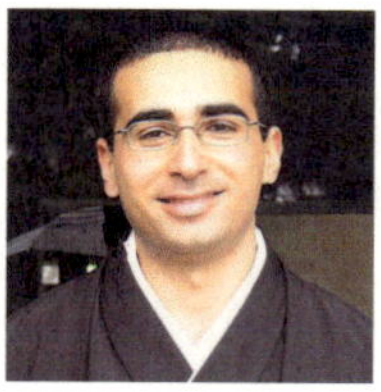

Dr. Ir. Haïtham Sghaier is an engineer in Biotechnology and professor (associate) of Radiation and Computational Biology at the National Center for Nuclear Sciences and Technology (CNSTN) in Tunisia. Dr. Sghaier has published on the evolution of ionizing-radiation-resistant Archaea and bacteria. Also, he has published on bioremediation issues. Currently, he is implicated in various ongoing sequencing projects and databases about Archaea and bacteria. In 2016, Dr. Sghaier won the TWAS Young Arab Scientist (YAS) Prize.

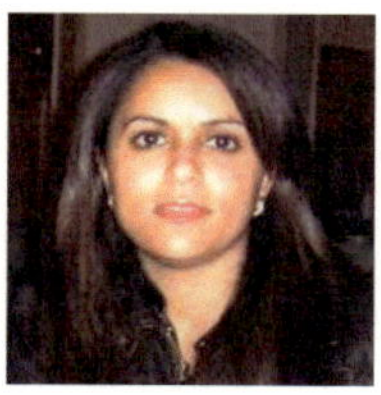

Dr. Afef Najjari is an assistant professor in Bioinformatics at the Faculty of Sciences of Tunisia, University of Tunis El Manar. Dr. Afef worked on several topics including genetic and enzymatic diversity of bacteria and microbial diversity in arid and saline ecosystems and mainly on archaeal groups. These works were funded by national and international projects. Currently, she is interested on metagenomic analysis, genome assemblies and annotations, transcriptomic data analysis (microarrays), and biological databases development.

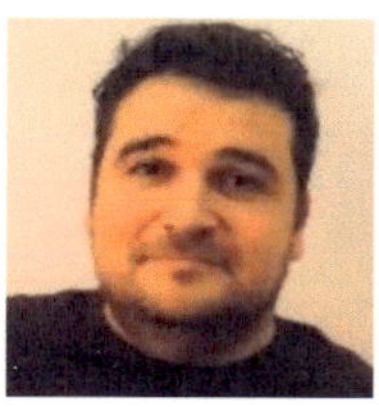

Dr. Kais Ghedira is an assistant professor in *Institut Pasteur de Tunis* (IPT) holding a PhD degree in bioinformatics. He has been involved in several international and national projects funded by European Commission, IPT, and NIH and is mainly involved in bioinformatics education and training in Africa. Dr. Ghedira is a bioinformatician with biological background. He is mainly interested in functional genomics and integrative biology, analysis of NGS high-throughput data (genome assembly, metagenomics), comparative genomics, gene expression (microarrays) and gene regulation analysis, and database and web tools development.

Contents

Preface

Members of the third domain of life, the Archaea, are not just germs and as such something to eradicate. Indeed, life could not exist without the functions and processes of these microorganisms. Presently, archaeal research is a mesmerizing, exciting, and growing field with potential impacts on biotechnology. Archaeal new biocatalysts and novel pharmaceuticals are expanding quickly for the benefits of humans.

This book presents a detailed portrait of many novel aspects related to archaeal biotechnology. In particular, it casts revealing light on the biotechnological applications of Euryarchaeota, archaeal potential next-generation probiotics, biocompounds from haloarchaea, a new tip based on the plasmid curing approach for improving the potential of thermophiles in various biotechnological applications.

We embarked upon this writing project to make pertinent contributions accessible to the scientific community. The editors hope that a large audience will enjoy reading and benefit from the chapters of this book entitled *Archaea: New Biocatalysts, Novel Pharmaceuticals, and Various Biotechnological Applications*.

Haïtham Sghaier
National Center for Nuclear Sciences and Technology,
Tunisia

Afef Najjari
Sidi Thabet Higher Institute for Biotechnology,
Tunisia

Kais Ghedira
Institut Pasteur de Tunis,
Tunisia

Chapter 1

Introductory Chapter: A Brief Overview of Archaeal Applications

Haïtham Sghaier, Afef Najjari and Kais Ghedira

Additional information is available at the end of the chapter

http://dx.doi.org/10.5772/intechopen.70289

1. Prologue

The first member of the Archaea was described in 1880 [1–3]. Yet, the recognition and formal description of the domain Archaea, as separated from Bacteria and Eukarya, occurred in 1977 during early phylogenetic analyses based upon ribosomal DNA sequences [4–6]. Indeed, members of the archaeal domain are characterized by several distinguishing traits [3] as confirmed later based on the first complete archaeal genome sequence obtained by Bult *et al.* [7] and the subsequent finished and ongoing archaeal sequencing projects (https://gold.jgi.doe.gov/organisms?Organism.Domain=ARCHAEAL, ftp://ftp.ncbi.nlm.nih.gov/genomes/refseq/archaea/) [8, 9].

The archaeal domain is composed of the **DPANN superphylum** [10]—*Aenigmarchaeota, Diapherotrites, Nanoarchaeota, Nanohaloarchaeota, Pacearchaeota, Parvarchaeota* and *Woesearchaeota* [11]—excluded from the common branch of the **TACK** (or TACKL [12]) **superphylum** [13]—*Aigarchaeota* [14], *Bathyarchaeota* [15], *Crenarchaeota* [16], *Korarchaeota* [17], *Lokiarchaeota* [18] and *Thaumarchaeota* [19]—with the **Euryarchaeota phylum** [16]—extreme halophilic Archaea, hyperthermephiles such as *Thermococcus* and *Pyrococcus*, most acidophilic-thermophilic prokaryotes, the thermophilic-acidophilic cell wall-less *Thermoplasma*, methanogens [20] and the Altiarchaeales clade [21].

The Archaea are ubiquitous in most terrestrial, aquatic and extreme environments (acidophilic, halophilic, mesophilic, methanogenic, psychrophilic and thermophilic) [20, 22]. Although very diversified with a great number of species, luckily, no member of the domain Archaea has been described as a pathogen for humans, animals or plants [23–25]. Thus, Archaea are a potentially valuable resource in the development of new biocatalysts, novel pharmaceuticals and various biotechnological applications. Applications of Archaea (for review, see [26–32] and references therein) may be subdivided into four main fields (**Figure 1**): (i) **commercial enzymes and/or molecules**, (ii) **environment**, (iii) **food** and (iv) **health**.

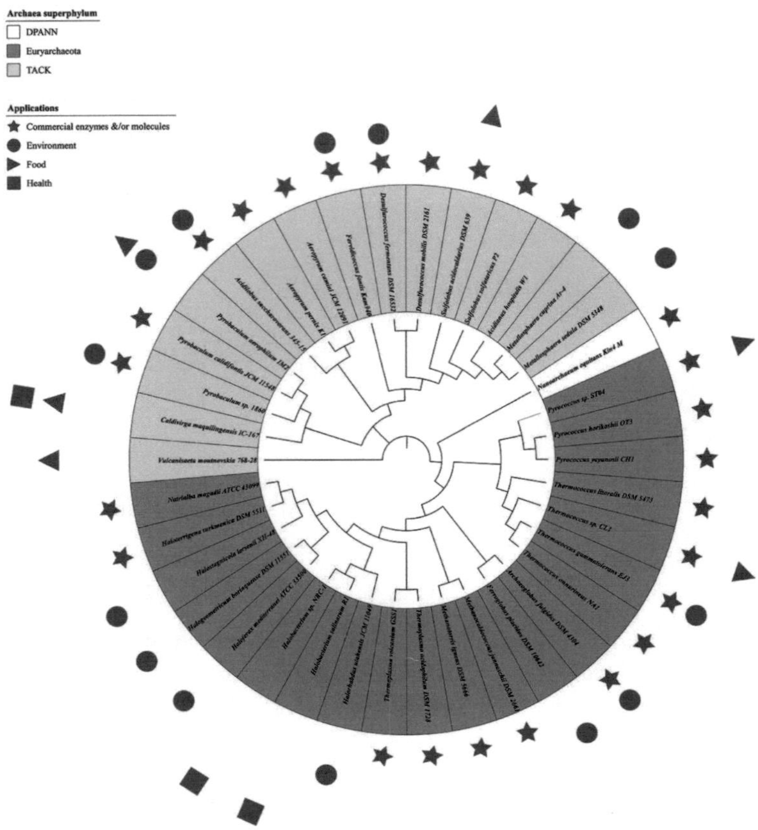

Figure 1. Examples of potential applications of Archaea in biotechnology depicted in a 16S rDNA phylogenetic tree visualized *via* the iTOL (Interactive Tree Of Life) tool [33]. Potential applications of Archaea were subdivided into four fields (commercial enzymes and/or molecules (stars), environment (circles), food (triangles) and health (squares)) based on the reference(s) listed following each species. Thirty eight (n=38) archaeal species were integrated into the above phylogenetic tree (one DPANN species (white color), 21 Euryarchaeota species (dark grey color), 16 TACK species (light grey color)): *Acidianus hospitalis* W1 (NC_015518) [34, 35], *Acidilobus saccharovorans* 345-15 (NC_014374) [36, 37], *Aeropyrum camini* JCM 12091 (NC_121692) [38], *Aeropyrum pernix* K1 (NC_000854) [39], *Archaeoglobus fulgidus* DSM 4304 (NC_000917) [40, 41], *Caldivirga maquilingensis* IC-167 (NC_009954) [42], *Desulfurococcus fermentans* DSM 16532 (NC_018001) [43], *Desulfurococcus mobilis* DSM 2161 (NC_014961) [44], *Ferroglobus placidus* DSM 10642 (NC_013849) [45], *Fervidicoccus fontis* Kam940 (NC_017461) [46], *Halobacterium salinarum* R1 (NC_010364) [47], *Halobacterium* sp. NRC-1 (NC_002607) [48], *Haloferax mediterranei* ATCC 33500 (NC_017941) [49], *Halogeometricum borinquense* DSM 11551 (NC_014729) [50], *Halorhabdus utahensis* JCM 11049 (NC_013158) [51], *Halostagnicola larsenii* XH-48 (NZ_CP007055) [52], *Haloterrigena turkmenica* DSM 5511 (NC_013743) [53], *Metallosphaera cuprina* Ar-4 (NC_015435) [54], *Metallosphaera sedula* DSM 5348 (NC_009440) [55], *Methanocaldococcus jannaschii* DSM 2661 (NC_000909) [27, 56], *Methanotorris igneus* DSM 5666 (NC_015562) [57], *Natrialba magadii* ATCC 43099 (NC_013922) [58], *Nanoarchaeum equitans* Kin4-M (NC_005213) [59, 60], *Pyrobaculum aerophilum* IM2 (NC_041958) [61, 62], *Pyrobaculum calidifontis* JCM 11548 (NC_009073) [63], *Pyrobaculum* sp. 1860 (NC_016645) [64, 65], *Pyrococcus horikoshii* OT3 (NC_000961) [66], *Pyrococcus* sp. ST04 (NC_017946) [67], *Pyrococcus yayanosii* CH1 (NC_015680) [68], *Sulfolobus acidocaldarius* DSM 639 (NC_007181) [69], *Sulfolobus solfataricus* P2 (NZ_LT549890) [70], *Thermococcus gammatolerans* EJ3 (NC_012804) [71], *Thermococcus litoralis* DSM 5473 (NC_022084) [72], *Thermococcus onnurineus* NA1 (NC_011529) [73], *Thermococcus* sp. CL1 (NC_018015) [74], *Thermoplasma acidophilum* DSM 1728 (NC_002578) [75, 76], *Thermoplasma volcanium* GSS1 (NC_002689) [77], *Vulcanisaeta moutnovskia* 768-28 (NC_015151) [78].

The book 'Archaea - New Biocatalysts, Novel Pharmaceuticals and Various Biotechnological Applications' contains five chapters.

The **first chapter** is an Introductory Chapter, where editors give a general overview of the content of the book.

The **second chapter** by Castro-Fernandez *et al.*, entitled 'Evolution, metabolism and molecular mechanisms underlying extreme adaptation of *Euryarchaeota* and its biotechnological potential', provides an interesting depiction of the phylum *Euryarchaeota* in terms of evolutive history, metabolic strategies, lipid composition, proteic structural adaptations and its biotechnological applications.

The **third chapter** 'Archaebiotics: archaea as pharmabiotics for treating chronic disease in humans?' was written by Ben Hania and co-authors. It promotes the idea that some specific archaea are potential next-generation probiotics.

The **fourth chapter** 'Biocompounds from haloarchaea and their uses in biotechnology' by Torregrosa-Crespo *et al.*, emphasizes the main characteristics of biocompounds from haloarchaea and their potential uses in biomedicine, pharmacy and industry.

The book concludes with a **(fifth) chapter** by Mizuno *et al.*, entitled 'Plasmid curing is a promising approach to improve thermophiles for biotechnological applications: perspectives in archaea', providing a new tip based on the plasmid-curing approach for improving the potential of thermophiles in various biotechnological applications.

Finally, we would like to thank all authors for their contributions. We are also grateful to InTech Publishing Process Managers, particularly Ms. Mirena Čalmić, Ms. Romina Rovan and Ms. Ana Pantar, who assisted us with patience until the publication of this book.

Author details

Haïtham Sghaier[1,2,3]*, Afef Najjari[3,4] and Kais Ghedira[4,5]

*Address all correspondence to: sghaier.haitham@gmail.com

1 Laboratory "Energy and Matter for Development of Nuclear Sciences" (LR16CNSTN02), National Center for Nuclear Sciences and Technology (CNSTN), Sidi Thabet, Tunisia

2 Laboratory "Biotechnology and Nuclear Technology" (LR16CNSTN01), CNSTN, Sidi Thabet, Tunisia

3 Univ. Manouba, ISBST, BVBGR-LR11ES31, Ariana, Tunisia

4 University of Tunis El Manar, Tunis, Tunisia

5 Laboratory of BioInformatics bioMathematics and bioStatistics (BIMS, LR16IPT09), Pasteur Institute of Tunis, Tunis, Tunisia

References

[1] Farlow WG. Part IV. Report for the commissioner. In: United States Commission of Fish and Fisheries. Washington DC: Government Printing Office; 1878. pp. 969-973. 1880

[2] Kocur M, Hodgkiss W. Taxonomic status of the genus *Halococcus* Schoop. International Journal of Systematic and Evolutionary Microbiology. 1973;**23**(2):151-156

[3] Cavicchioli R. Archaea—timeline of the third domain. Nature Reviews Microbiology. 2011;**9**(1):51-61

[4] Balch WE, Magrum LJ, Fox GE, Wolfe RS, Woese CR. An ancient divergence among the bacteria. Journal of Molecular Evolution. 1977;**9**(4):305-311

[5] Fox GE, Magrum LJ, Balch WE, Wolfe RS, Woese CR. Classification of methanogenic bacteria by 16S ribosomal RNA characterization. Proceedings of the National Academy of Sciences of the United States of America. 1977;**74**(10):4537-4541

[6] Woese CR, Fox GE. Phylogenetic structure of the prokaryotic domain: The primary kingdoms. Proceedings of the National Academy of Sciences of the United States of America. 1977;**74**(11):5088-5090

[7] Bult CJ, White O, Olsen GJ, Zhou L, Fleischmann RD, Sutton GG, Blake JA, FitzGerald LM, Clayton RA, Gocayne JD, et al. Complete genome sequence of the methanogenic archaeon, *Methanococcus jannaschii*. Science. 1996;**273**(5278):1058-1073

[8] Reddy TB, Thomas AD, Stamatis D, Bertsch J, Isbandi M, Jansson J, Mallajosyula J, Pagani I, Lobos EA, Kyrpides NC. The Genomes OnLine Database (GOLD) v.5: A metadata management system based on a four level (meta)genome project classification. Nucleic Acids Research. 2015;**43**(Database issue):D1099-D1106

[9] Tatusova T, Ciufo S, Fedorov B, O'Neill K, Tolstoy I. RefSeq microbial genomes database: New representation and annotation strategy. Nucleic Acids Research. 2014;**42**(Database issue):D553-D559

[10] Rinke C, Schwientek P, Sczyrba A, Ivanova NN, Anderson IJ, Cheng JF, Darling A, Malfatti S, Swan BK, Gies EA, et al: Insights into the phylogeny and coding potential of microbial dark matter. Nature. 2013;**499**(7459):431-437

[11] Castelle CJ, Wrighton KC, Thomas BC, Hug LA, Brown CT, Wilkins MJ, Frischkorn KR, Tringe SG, Singh A, Markillie LM, et al. Genomic expansion of domain archaea highlights roles for organisms from new phyla in anaerobic carbon cycling. Current Biology: CB. 2015;**25**(6):690-701

[12] Da Cunha V, Gaia M, Gadelle D, Nasir A, Forterre P. Lokiarchaea are close relatives of Euryarchaeota, not bridging the gap between prokaryotes and eukaryotes. PLoS Genetics. 2017;**13**(6):e1006810

[13] Guy L, Ettema TJ. The archaeal 'TACK' superphylum and the origin of eukaryotes. Trends in Microbiology. 2011;**19**(12):580-587

[14] Nunoura T, Takaki Y, Kakuta J, Nishi S, Sugahara J, Kazama H, Chee GJ, Hattori M, Kanai A, Atomi H, et al. Insights into the evolution of Archaea and eukaryotic protein modifier systems revealed by the genome of a novel archaeal group. Nucleic Acids Research. 2011;**39**(8):3204-3223

[15] Meng J, Xu J, Qin D, He Y, Xiao X, Wang F. Genetic and functional properties of uncultivated MCG archaea assessed by metagenome and gene expression analyses. The ISME Journal. 2014;**8**(3):650-659

[16] Woese CR, Kandler O, Wheelis ML. Towards a natural system of organisms: Proposal for the domains Archaea, Bacteria, and Eucarya. Proceedings of the National Academy of Sciences of the United States of America. 1990;**87**(12):4576-4579

[17] Barns SM, Delwiche CF, Palmer JD, Pace NR. Perspectives on archaeal diversity, thermophily and monophyly from environmental rRNA sequences. Proceedings of the National Academy of Sciences of the United States of America. 1996;**93**(17):9188-9193

[18] Spang A, Saw JH, Jorgensen SL, Zaremba-Niedzwiedzka K, Martijn J, Lind AE, van Eijk R, Schleper C, Guy L, Ettema TJ. Complex archaea that bridge the gap between prokaryotes and eukaryotes. Nature. 2015;**521**(7551):173-179

[19] Brochier-Armanet C, Boussau B, Gribaldo S, Forterre P. Mesophilic Crenarchaeota: Proposal for a third archaeal phylum, the Thaumarchaeota. Nature Reviews Microbiology. 2008;**6**(3):245-252

[20] Amils R. Euryarchaeota. In: Gargaud M, Irvine WM, Amils R, Cleaves HJ, Pinti DL, Quintanilla JC, Rouan D, Spohn T, Tirard S, Viso M, editors. Encyclopedia of Astrobiology Berlin, Heidelberg: Springer Berlin Heidelberg; 2015. pp. 764-765

[21] Probst AJ, Moissl-Eichinger C. "*Altiarchaeales*": Uncultivated archaea from the subsurface. Life. 2015;**5**(2):1381-1395

[22] Ferrera I, Takacs-Vesbach CD, Reysenbach A-L. Archaeal ecology. In: Encyclopedia of Life Sciences (ELS). Chichester: John Wiley & Sons, Ltd; 2008. DOI: 10.1002/9780470015902.a9780470000338.pub9780470015902

[23] Cavicchioli R, Curmi PM, Saunders N, Thomas T. Pathogenic archaea: Do they exist? BioEssays: News and Reviews in Molecular, Cellular and Developmental Biology. 2003;**25**(11):1119-1128

[24] Reeve JN. Archaebacteria Then ... Archaes Now (Are There Really No Archaeal Pathogens?). Journal of Bacteriology. 1999;**181**(12):3613-3617

[25] Aminov RI. Role of archaea in human disease. Frontiers in Cellular and Infection Microbiology. 2013;**3**:42

[26] Schiraldi C, Giuliano M, De Rosa M. Perspectives on biotechnological applications of archaea. Archaea. 2002;**1**(2):75-86

[27] Eichler J. Biotechnological uses of archaeal extremozymes. Biotechnology Advances. 2001;**19**(4):261-278

[28] Reed CJ, Lewis H, Trejo E, Winston V, Evilia C. Protein adaptations in archaeal extremophiles. Archaea. 2013;**2013**:373275

[29] Litchfield CD. Potential for industrial products from the halophilic Archaea. Journal of Industrial Microbiology and Biotechnology. 2011;**38**(10):1635-1647

[30] Egorova K, Antranikian G. Industrial relevance of thermophilic Archaea. Current Opinion in Microbiology. 2005;**8**(6):649-655

[31] Dumorne K, Cordova DC, Astorga-Elo M, Renganathan P. Extremozymes: A potential source for industrial applications. Journal of Microbiology and Biotechnology. 2017;**27**(4):649-659

[32] Antunes A, Simões MF, Grötzinger SW, Eppinger J, Bragança J, Bajic VB. Bioprospecting Archaea: Focus on extreme halophiles. In: Paterson R, Lima N, editors. Bioprospecting: Success, Potential and Constraints. Cham: Springer International Publishing; 2017. pp. 81-112

[33] Letunic I, Bork P. Interactive tree of life (iTOL) v3: An online tool for the display and annotation of phylogenetic and other trees. Nucleic Acids Research. 2016;**44**(W1):W242-W245

[34] You X, Zhang Q, Zheng H, Jiang C. Adaptation of *Acidianus hospitalis* W1 to oligotrophic and acidic hot spring environments. Wei Sheng Wu Xue Bao = Acta Microbiologica Sinica. 2014;**54**(10):1193-1203

[35] Krupovic M, Peixeiro N, Bettstetter M, Rachel R, Prangishvili D. Archaeal tetrathionate hydrolase goes viral: Secretion of a sulfur metabolism enzyme in the form of virus-like particles. Applied and Environmental Microbiology. 2012;**78**(15):5463-5465

[36] Gumerov VM, Rakitin AL, Mardanov AV, Ravin NV. A novel highly thermostable multifunctional beta-glycosidase from crenarchaeon *Acidilobus saccharovorans*. Archaea. 2015;2015:978632

[37] Mardanov AV, Svetlitchnyi VA, Beletsky AV, Prokofeva MI, Bonch-Osmolovskaya EA, Ravin NV, Skryabin KG. The genome sequence of the crenarchaeon *Acidilobus saccharovorans* supports a new order, Acidilobales, and suggests an important ecological role in terrestrial acidic hot springs. Applied and Environmental Microbiology. 2010;**76**(16):5652-5657

[38] Nishimura H, Sako Y. Purification and characterization of the oxygen-thermostable hydrogenase from the aerobic hyperthermophilic archaeon *Aeropyrum camini*. Journal of Bioscience and Bioengineering. 2009;**108**(4):299-303

[39] Mino K, Ishikawa K. Characterization of a novel thermostable O-acetylserine sulfhydrylase from *Aeropyrum pernix* K1. Journal of Bacteriology. 2003;**185**(7):2277-2284

[40] Beblo-Vranesevic KA-Ohoo, Galinski EA, Rachel R, Huber H, Rettberg P. Influence of osmotic stress on desiccation and irradiation tolerance of (hyper)-thermophilic microorganisms. Archives of Microbiology. 2017;**199**(1):17-28

[41] Toso DB, Javed MM, Czornyj E, Gunsalus RA-O, Zhou ZH. Discovery and characterization of iron sulfide and polyphosphate bodies coexisting in *Archaeoglobus fulgidus cells. Archaea*. 2016. DOI: 10.1155/2016/4706532

[42] Letsididi R, Hassanin HA, Koko MY, Ndayishimiye JB, Zhang T, Jiang B, Stressler T, Fischer L, Mu W. Characterization of a thermostable glycoside hydrolase (CMbg0408) from the hyperthermophilic archaeon *Caldivirga maquilingensis* IC-167. Journal of the Science of Food and Agriculture. 2017;**97**(7):2132-2140

[43] Susanti D, Johnson EF, Rodriguez JR, Anderson I, Perevalova AA, Kyrpides N, Lucas S, Han J, Lapidus A, Cheng JF, et al. Complete genome sequence of *Desulfurococcus fermentans*, a hyperthermophilic cellulolytic crenarchaeon isolated from a freshwater hot spring in Kamchatka, Russia. Journal of Bacteriology. 2012;**194**(20):5703-5704

[44] Susanti D, Johnson EF, Lapidus A, Han J, Reddy TB, Pilay M, Ivanova NN, Markowitz VM, Woyke T, Kyrpides NC, et al. Permanent draft genome sequence of *Desulfurococcus mobilis* type strain DSM 2161, a thermoacidophilic sulfur-reducing crenarchaeon isolated from acidic hot springs of Hveravellir, Iceland. Standards in Genomic Sciences. 2016;**11**:3

[45] Aklujkar M, Risso C, Smith J, Beaulieu D, Dubay R, Giloteaux L, DiBurro K, Holmes D. Anaerobic degradation of aromatic amino acids by the hyperthermophilic archaeon *Ferroglobus placidus*. Microbiology. 2014;**160**(Pt 12):2694-2709

[46] Lebedinsky AV, Mardanov AV, Kublanov IV, Gumerov VM, Beletsky AV, Perevalova AA, Bidzhieva S, Bonch-Osmolovskaya EA, Skryabin KG, Ravin NV: Analysis of the complete genome of *Fervidococcus fontis* confirms the distinct phylogenetic position of the order *Fervidicoccales* and suggests its environmental function. Extremophiles. 2014;**18**(2):295-309

[47] Cherin E, Melis JM, Bourdeau RW, Yin M, Kochmann DM, Foster FS, Shapiro MG. Acoustic behavior of *Halobacterium salinarum* gas vesicles in the high-frequency range: Experiments and modeling. Ultrasound in Medicine & Biology. 2017;**43**(5):1016-1030

[48] Balakrishnan A, DasSarma P, Bhattacharjee O, Kim JM, DasSarma S, Chakravortty D. Halobacterial nano vesicles displaying murine bactericidal permeability-increasing protein rescue mice from lethal endotoxic shock. Scientific Reports. 2016;**6**:33679

[49] Alsafadi D, Al-Mashaqbeh O. A one-stage cultivation process for the production of poly-3-(hydroxybutyrate-co-hydroxyvalerate) from olive mill wastewater by *Haloferax mediterranei*. New Biotechnology. 2017;**34**:47-53

[50] Salgaonkar BB, Braganca JM. Biosynthesis of poly(3-hydroxybutyrate-co-3-hydroxyvalerate) by *Halogeometricum borinquense* strain E3. International Journal of Biological Macromolecules. 2015;**78**:339-346

[51] Anderson I, Tindall BJ, Pomrenke H, Goker M, Lapidus A, Nolan M, Copeland A, Glavina Del Rio T, Chen F, Tice H, et al. Complete genome sequence of *Halorhabdus utahensis* type strain (AX-2). Standards in Genomic Sciences. 2009;**1**(3):218-225

[52] Kanekar PP, Kulkarni SO, Kanekar SP, Shouche Y, Jani K, Sharma A. Exploration of a haloarchaeon, *Halostagnicola larsenii,* isolated from rock pit sea water, West Coast of Maharashtra, India, for the production of bacteriorhodopsin. Journal of Applied Microbiology. 2016;**120**(4):1136

[53] Squillaci G, Finamore R, Diana P, Restaino OF, Schiraldi C, Arbucci S, Ionata E, La Cara F, Morana A. Production and properties of an exopolysaccharide synthesized by the extreme halophilic archaeon *Haloterrigena turkmenica*. Applied Microbiology and Biotechnology. 2016;**100**(2):613-623

[54] Liu LJ, You XY, Zheng H, Wang S, Jiang CY, Liu SJ. Complete genome sequence of *Metallosphaera cuprina,* a metal sulfide-oxidizing archaeon from a hot spring. Journal of Bacteriology. 2011;**193**(13):3387-3388

[55] Artz JH, White SN, Zadvornyy OA, Fugate CJ, Hicks D, Gauss GH, Posewitz MC, Boyd ES, Peters JW. Biochemical and structural properties of a thermostable mercuric ion reductase from *Metallosphaera sedula*. Frontiers in Bioengineering and Biotechnology. 2015;**3**:97

[56] Kim JW, Flowers LO, Whiteley M, Peeples TL. Biochemical confirmation and characterization of the family-57-like alpha-amylase of *Methanococcus jannaschii*. Folia Microbiologica. 2001;**46**(6):467-473

[57] Hei DJ, Clark DS. Pressure stabilization of proteins from extreme thermophiles. Applied and Environmental Microbiology. 1994;**60**(3):932-939

[58] Polosina YY, Zamyatkin DF, Kostyukova AS, Filimonov VV, Fedorov OV. Stability of *Natrialba magadii* NDP kinase: Comparisons with other halophilic proteins. Extremophiles. 2002;**6**(2):135-142

[59] Waters E, Hohn MJ, Ahel I, Graham DE, Adams MD, Barnstead M, Beeson KY, Bibbs L, Bolanos R, Keller M, et al. The genome of *Nanoarchaeum equitans*: Insights into early archaeal evolution and derived parasitism. Proceedings of the National Academy of Sciences of the United States of America. 2003;**100**(22):12984-12988

[60] Olszewski M, Balsewicz J, Nowak M, Maciejewska N, Cyranka-Czaja A, Zalewska-Piątek B, Piątek R, Kur J. Characterization of a single-stranded DNA-binding-like protein from *Nanoarchaeum equitans*—A nucleic acid binding protein with broad substrate specificity. PLOS ONE. 2015;**10**(5):e0126563

[61] Kaper T, Talik B, Ettema TJ, Bos H, van der Maarel MJ, Dijkhuizen L. Amylomaltase of *Pyrobaculum aerophilum* IM2 produces thermoreversible starch gels. Applied and Environmental Microbiology. 2005;**71**(9):5098-5106

[62] de Vries S, Momcilovic M, Strampraad MJ, Whitelegge JP, Baghai A, Schroder I. Adaptation to a high-tungsten environment: *Pyrobaculum aerophilum* contains an active tungsten nitrate reductase. Biochemistry. 2010;**49**(45):9911-9921

[63] Satomura T, Zhang XD, Hara Y, Doi K, Sakuraba H, Ohshima T: Characterization of a novel dye-linked L-proline dehydrogenase from an aerobic hyperthermophilic archaeon, *Pyrobaculum calidifontis*. Applied Microbiology and Biotechnology. 2011; **89**(4):1075-1082

[64] Shao H, Xu L, Yan Y. Biochemical characterization of a carboxylesterase from the archaeon *Pyrobaculum* sp. 1860 and a rational explanation of its substrate specificity and thermostability. International Journal of Molecular Sciences. 2014;**15**(9):16885-16910

[65] Mardanov AV, Gumerov VM, Slobodkina GB, Beletsky AV, Bonch-Osmolovskaya EA, Ravin NV, Skryabin KG. Complete genome sequence of strain 1860, a crenarchaeon of the genus *Pyrobaculum* able to grow with various electron acceptors. Journal of Bacteriology. 2012;**194**(3):727-728

[66] Ishikawa K, Ishida H, Matsui I, Kawarabayasi Y, Kikuchi H. Novel bifunctional hyperthermostable carboxypeptidase/aminoacylase from *Pyrococcus horikoshii* OT3. Applied and Environmental Microbiology. 2001;**67**(2):673-679

[67] Jung JH, Seo DH, Holden JF, Park CS. Maltose-forming alpha-amylase from the hyperthermophilic archaeon *Pyrococcus* sp. ST04. Applied Microbiology and Biotechnology. 2014;**98**(5):2121-2131

[68] Fu L, Li X, Xiao X, Xu J. Purification and characterization of a thermostable aliphatic amidase from the hyperthermophilic archaeon *Pyrococcus yayanosii* CH1. Extremophiles. 2014;**18**(2):429-440

[69] Pennacchio A, Sannino V, Sorrentino G, Rossi M, Raia CA, Esposito L. Biochemical and structural characterization of recombinant short-chain NAD(H)-dependent dehydrogenase/reductase from *Sulfolobus acidocaldarius* highly enantioselective on diaryl diketone benzil. Applied Microbiology and Biotechnology. 2013;**97**(9):3949-3964

[70] Zhu S, Huang R, Gao S, Li X, Zheng G. Discovery and characterization of a second extremely thermostable (+)-gamma-lactamase from *Sulfolobus solfataricus* P2. Journal of Bioscience and Bioengineering. 2016;**121**(5):484-490

[71] Jolivet E, L'Haridon S, Corre E, Forterre P, Prieur D. *Thermococcus gammatolerans* sp. nov., a hyperthermophilic archaeon from a deep-sea hydrothermal vent that resists ionizing radiation. International Journal of Systematic and Evolutionary Microbiology. 2003;**53**(Pt 3):847-851

[72] Washio T, Kato S, Oikawa T. Molecular cloning and enzymological characterization of pyridoxal 5′-phosphate independent aspartate racemase from hyperthermophilic archaeon *Thermococcus litoralis* DSM 5473. Extremophiles. 2016;**20**(5):711-721

[73] Kim YJ, Lee HS, Kwon ST, Lee JH, Kang SG. Enhancing the processivity of a family B-type DNA polymerase of *Thermococcus onnurineus* and application to long PCR. Biotechnology Letters. 2014;**36**(5):985-992

[74] Jeon EJ, Jung JH, Seo DH, Jung DH, Holden JF, Park CS. Bioinformatic and biochemical analysis of a novel maltose-forming alpha-amylase of the GH57 family in the hyperthermophilic archaeon *Thermococcus* sp. CL1. Enzyme and Microbial Technology. 2014;**60**:9-15

[75] Kim JH, Sung MW, Lee EH, Nam KH, Hwang KY. Crystallization and preliminary X-ray diffraction analysis of 5,10-methylenetetrahydrofolate dehydrogenase/cyclohydrolase from *Thermoplasma acidophilum* DSM 1728. Journal of Microbiology and Biotechnology. 2008;**18**(2):283-286

[76] Kim YK, Mizutani K, Rhee KH, Nam KH, Lee WH, Lee EH, Kim EE, Park SY, Hwang KY. Structural and mutational analysis of tRNA intron-splicing endonuclease from *Thermoplasma acidophilum* DSM 1728: Catalytic mechanism of tRNA intron-splicing endonucleases. Journal of Bacteriology. 2007;**189**(22):8339-8346

[77] Kocabiyik S, Demirok B. Cloning and overexpression of a thermostable signal peptide peptidase (SppA) from *Thermoplasma volcanium* GSS1 in E. coli. Biotechnology Journal. 2009;**4**(7):1055-1065

[78] Gumerov VM, Mardanov AV, Beletsky AV, Prokofeva MI, Bonch-Osmolovskaya EA, Ravin NV, Skryabin KG. Complete genome sequence of "*Vulcanisaeta moutnovskia*" strain 768-28, a novel member of the hyperthermophilic crenarchaeal genus *Vulcanisaeta*. Journal of Bacteriology. 2011;**193**(9):2355-2356

Chapter 2

Evolution, Metabolism and Molecular Mechanisms Underlying Extreme Adaptation of *Euryarchaeota* and Its Biotechnological Potential

Victor Castro-Fernandez, Ricardo Zamora, Alejandra Herrera-Morande, Gabriel Vallejos, Felipe Gonzalez-Ordenes and Victoria Guixé

Additional information is available at the end of the chapter

http://dx.doi.org/10.5772/intechopen.69943

Abstract

Archaeal organisms harbor many unique genotypic and phenotypic properties, testifying their peculiar evolutionary status. Thus, the so-called extremophiles must be adequately adapted to cope with many extreme environments with regard to metabolic processes, biological functions, genomes, and transcriptomes to overcome the challenges of life. This chapter will illustrate recent progress in the research on extremophiles from the phylum *Euryarchaeota* and compile their evolutive history, metabolic strategies, lipid composition, the structural adaptations of their enzymes to temperature, salinity, and pH and their biotechnological applications. Archaeal organisms have evolved to deal with one or more extreme conditions, and over the evolution, they have accumulated changes in order to optimize protein structure and enzyme activity. The structural basis of these adaptations resulted in the construction of a vast repertoire of macromolecules with particular features not found in other organisms. This repertoire can be explored as an inexhaustible source of biological molecules for industrial or biotechnological applications. We hope that the information compiled herein will open new research lines that will shed light on various aspects of these extremophilic microorganisms. In addition, this information will be a valuable resource for future studies looking for archaeal enzymes with particular properties.

Keywords: archaea, archaea evolution, archaeal lipids, archaea metabolism, biotechnological applications, methanogenesis, *Euryarchaeota*, extremozymes

1. Introduction

Archaea represents the third domain of life. Their peculiar evolutionary status conforms to their unique genotypic and phenotypic properties. Except for methanogenesis, which has not yet been described in bacteria, all central metabolic pathways discovered in archaea also exist in bacteria, although in some cases with important and novel modifications. Archaeal organisms can be either heterotrophs or autotrophs (chemio- or photo-lithoautotroph) and can use a large variety of electron donors and acceptors [1]. One of the most striking features of archaea organisms is their relation with hyperthermophilicity as they are able to colonize ecological niches even above 95°C. This property relies in part on the unique structure of archaeal lipids, which are able to maintain impermeability of the cytoplasmic membrane to ions at such high temperatures. Although archaea are often believed to live in extreme environments, they can also be found in many diverse locations including even moderate environmental conditions.

The phylum *Euryarchaeota*, in archaea, comprises an extremely physiologically diverse group of microorganisms, adapted to the most extreme environments known so far. This phylum includes organisms adapted to different temperature niches (thermophiles, mesophiles, and psychrophiles), pH (acidophiles), and the organisms those grow at elevated salt concentrations (halophiles). On the other hand, the phylum, *Crenarchaeota*, comprises a much more limited phenotypic diversity of cultivable organisms. This chapter focuses on the phylum *Euryarchaeota* and considering the industrial potential of their proteins.

2. The *Euryarchaeota* phylogenetic tree

The evolutionary studies of archaea are important for understanding the origin of life and the course of evolution of the organisms that populate the earth. In the 1970s, Carl Woese's work showed that RNA of the small subunit of the ribosome (SSU rRNA) could be used to define phylogenetic relationships, which allowed the construction of a universal tree of life [2]. From these studies emerged the discovery of archaea, demonstrating that living organisms on earth can be divided into three domains (archaea, eukarya, and bacteria). Initially, two phyla were identified in archaea: *Crenarchaeota* and *Euryarchaeota* [3]. Subsequently, new phyla, namely *Korarchaeota, Nanoarchaeota,* and *Thaumarchaeota,* were proposed based on SSU rRNA [2].

The phylum *Euryarchaeota* comprises an extreme physiologically diverse group of microorganisms, adapted to the most extreme environments known. The members constitute the greatest phenotypic diversity among the cultivable species known to date, including halophiles, methanogens, some thermoacidophiles, and some hyperthermophiles. Through SSU rRNA, the following orders of *Euryarchaeota* were identified: *Thermococcales, Methanobacteriales, Methanococcales, Thermoplasmatales, Halobacteriales, Methanosarcinales, Methanomicrobiales, Methanocellales,* and *Archaeoglobales.*

However, at the end of the 1990s, the phylogenies based on SSU rRNA were questioned regarding their ability to reconstruct the more ancestral speciation events, given the lack of a phylogenetic signal [4]. The phylogenetic trees, reconstructed with SSU rRNA by maximum likelihood and evaluated by bootstrap (a method to evaluate the robustness of nodes in a tree), showed that the most ancestral nodes of the phylum *Euryarchaeota* have '60% statistical significance, which makes difficult to have confidence in the phylogenetic relationship between the different orders. Then, by using SSU rRNA, the orders that diverge first and those that diverge last cannot be established [5].

The evolutionary relationships among the archaea orders have been established by the sequencing of several genomes. Petitjean et al. [6] identified 200 protein families, along with 57 ribosomal proteins and 14 RNA polymerase subunits, which represent 273 phylogenetic markers in 129 archaeal genomes. With this conserved core of archaeal genes, they inferred the phylogeny of the nodes of different orders with high robustness (statistical significance >95%). The tree topology obtained with this core of proteins is generally consistent with other topologies such as that obtained by Battistuzzia and Hedgesa [7].

The topology of these phylogenies shows that *Thermococcales* were the first group to diverge (**Figure 1**) in *Euryarchaeota*, approximately 3594 Ma ago, ruling out the possibility that methanogenesis was an ancestral metabolic process in the *Euryarchaeota*. Subsequently, the orders *Methanopyrales*, *Methanobacteriales*, and *Methanococcales* diverged around 3468 Ma ago, and methanogens class I or *Methanomada* appeared [6]. Later on, the order *Thermoplasmatales* diverged (3160 Ma ago), followed by the order *Archaeoglobales* (2799 Ma ago). Finally, methanogens class II diverged (*Methanocellales*, *Methanosarcinales*, and *Methanomicrobiales*), and from this group, the order *Halobacteriales* emerged [6]. However, this hypothesis is debatable as in some topologies, *Halobacteriales* appear prior to the divergence of methanogens class II [7].

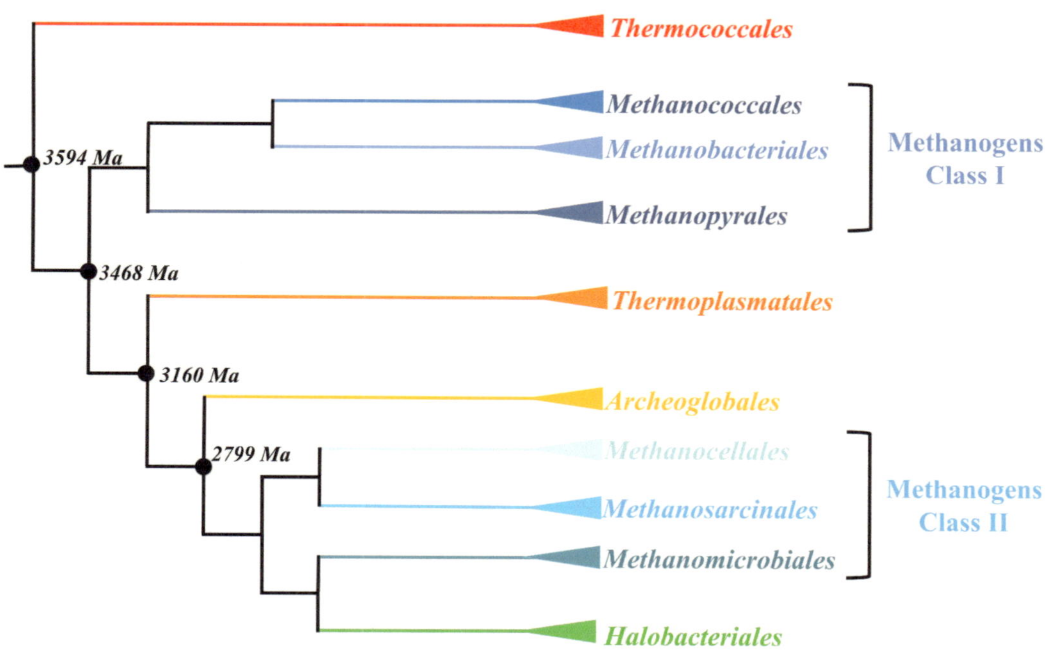

Figure 1. Schematic representation of phylogenetic relationships between the orders of *Euryarchaeota*. The estimated time in millions of years (Ma) for the divergence of some orders is shown according to the time-tree [7].

3. *Euryarchaeota* metabolism

Euryarchaeota organisms show very diverse metabolism. For example, phylogenetically close orders can exhibit very different kinds of metabolism, while important similarities can be observed in distantly related orders. Most of the *Euryarchaeota* are strictly anaerobic, although some of them can grow at low oxygen concentrations. *Euryarchaeota,* like most of the anaerobic organisms studied, lacks the defense mechanisms against oxidative stress (ROS). However, recently, the ability of *P. furiosus* to grow even in the presence of 8% oxygen has been described, which led to postulate the existence of a mechanism through which a part of the electrons destined to H_2 production are diverted to the O_2 reduction [8]. Further, this phylum comprises mainly autotrophic organisms, and some heterotrophs can be found. This trait has been suggested to be an evolutive novelty acquired later [9].

The systematic studies of archaeal metabolism were undertaken soon after the first genome sequence from archaea was obtained. The initial studies contemplated metabolic reconstructions based on the presence of homologous sequences with known activities [10]. In parallel, the *in vitro* studies with cellular cultures that included metabolite and enzymatic measurements in crude extracts began to appear. The most of our current knowledge about their metabolism has been derived from the exhaustive studies performed with the model organisms like *Methanocaldococcus jannaschii* (the first archaeal genome to be sequenced), *Methanococcus maripaludis* [11] (order *Methanococcales*), *Methanosarcina acetivorans* [12] (order *Methanosarcinales*), *Thermococcus kodakarensis*, and *P. furiosus* [13] (both from order *Thermococcales*)—just to mention some of them. In **Figure 2**, a simplified scheme showing the main metabolic pathways of the archaeal life is presented, using *Thermococcales*, *Methanococcales*, and *Methanosarcinales* as examples.

Heterotrophs from *Thermococcales* are the most studied organisms, which can be grown in different conditions using sugars, peptides, or polysaccharides as a carbon source [14, 15]. In these organisms, glycolysis or the Embden-Meyerhof pathway (EM) plays a fundamental role in the production of reduced equivalents and ATP [16]. In this pathway, important modifications to the traditional glycolysis can be observed, such as the phosphorylation of glucose and fructose-6-P is performed by a glucokinase (ADP-GK) and a phosphofructokinase (ADP-PFK) employing ADP instead of ATP as a phosphoryl donor [17, 18], and the canonical G3PDH is replaced by a glyceraldehyde-3-phosphate ferredoxin oxidoreductase (GAPOR) [19]. In addition, a pyruvate ferredoxin oxidoreductase (POR) that decarboxylases pyruvate to synthesize Acetyl-CoA is also present in these organisms [20]. In both the aforementioned reactions, reduced ferredoxin is produced, which constitutes one of the most important electron carriers. Ferredoxin produced in glycolysis is oxidized later by a membrane hydrogenase, coupled to molecular hydrogen production [21]. During this process, a proton is exported to the extracellular medium, contributing to the proton gradient which in turn allows ATP production carried out by the ATP synthase enzyme [21]. Alternatively, archaea possess a unique Acetyl-CoA synthetase able to synthesize acetate from Acetyl-CoA coupled to ATP production [22]. This reaction, along with pyruvate synthesis by pyruvate kinase, is the only step where phosphorylation of ADP at a substrate level occurs in glycolysis. In these organisms, as well as the autotrophs belonging to *Euryarchaeota*, the presence of an incomplete reductive Kreb's cycle

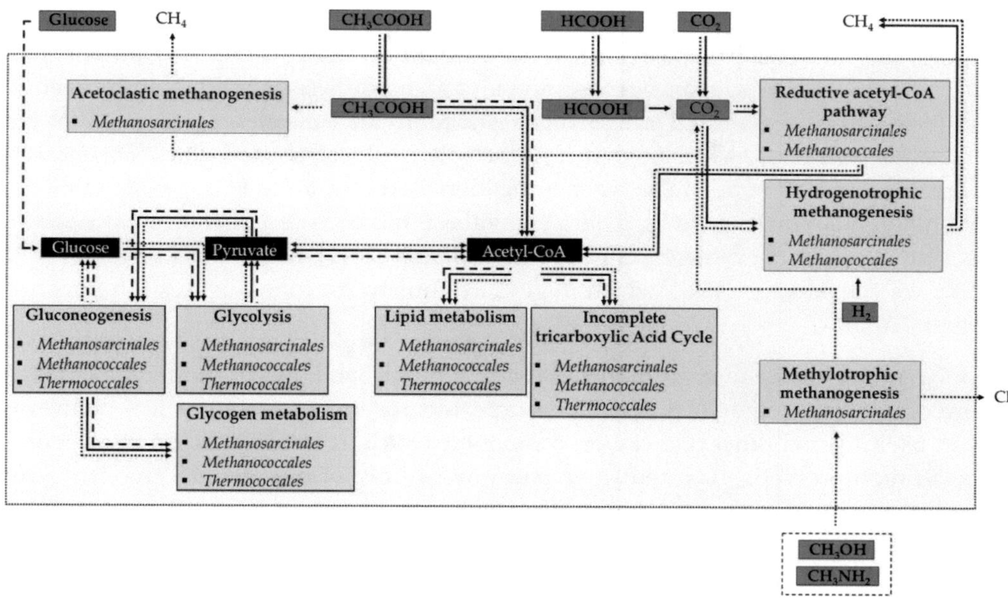

Figure 2. The simplied scheme of *Euryarchaeal* metabolism. *Thermococcales* are used as an example to represent heterotrophic archaea, *Methanococcales* as an example of class I methanogens and *Methanosarcinales* of class II methanogens. Light gray squares represent main metabolic processes mentioned in the text. The genera carrying each process are enclosed in a square. The relevant metabolites that can enter the cell are represented in dark gray squares. Metabolites that serve as intermediaries and connecting different processes are represented by black squares. CH_4, one of the major metabolic final products from methanogenic archaea is shown. The arrows represent connections between metabolites and metabolic processes. The dashed arrows represent the pathways present in *Thermococcales*; the black arrows represent the pathways present in *Methanococcales*, and the dotted arrows represent the pathways present in *Methanosarcinales*.

has been reported and it has been postulated that its function is the production of metabolic intermediates for amino acid synthesis and other anabolic processes [23].

Thermococcales can use elemental sulfur as the final electron acceptor producing sulfhydric acid as a final metabolic product [14]. However, in most cases, the presence of sulfur is not necessary, and alternatively, molecular hydrogen is produced as the final metabolic product [24]. This reaction is mainly carried out by a ferredoxin-dependent membrane hydrogenase. In the presence of elemental sulfur, the expression of this hydrogenase is diminished with the concomitant decrease in H_2 production. Under these conditions, ferredoxin is oxidized by a membrane oxidoreductase coupled to NADPH production and H^+ ions are exported to the extracellular medium. Later, an NADPH-dependent oxidoreductase reduces elemental sulfur, producing sulfhydric acid [24].

In autotrophic organisms of *Euryarchaeota*, such as methanogens class I (*Methanococcales*) and methanogens class II (*Methanosarcinales*), glycolysis also shows certain modifications; of them, most are shared with *Thermococcales* [16]. However, important differences can be observed in *Methanococcales*; since these organisms lack the ADP-GK gene, the ADP-PFK enzyme performs both phosphorylating activities at the same active site [25, 26]. It has been postulated that in both classes of methanogens, glycolysis is a secondary pathway since during the growth in the presence of a suitable amount of nutrients these organisms maintain active pathways like gluconeogenesis and glycogen synthesis [12, 27]. In the absence of nutrients, glycolysis is activated as a salvage route to produce metabolic intermediates and substrates for methanogenesis. Nonetheless, the role of glycolysis and gluconeogenesis in these organisms is still under an active investigation. Recently, an ADP-dependent PFK-GK with more catalytic efficiency toward glucose synthesis has been described in *M. maripaludis*, but its physiological relevance has not been elucidated [26]. Further, both activities (PFK and GK) are activated by AMP, which might have important consequences for glycolysis regulation [26].

Methanogens are unable to grow in the presence of sugars, peptides or compounds of three or more carbons since they lack specific transporters for these substances [28]. However, they can use CO_2 and other one-carbon compounds, such as formate, as a carbon source. Carbon fixation proceeds via a reductive pathway of Acetyl-CoA (Wood-Ljungdahl pathway) where two molecules of CO_2 are reduced and one molecule of Acetyl-CoA is produced [29]. This reduction is carried out by the oxidation of two equivalents of ferredoxin and one equivalent of coenzyme F420 (a unique coenzyme from methanogenic organisms) [30]. The methanogens, by using the POR enzyme, carry out the carboxylation of Acetyl-CoA to form pyruvate and, in this way, generate the substrates for gluconeogenesis or amino acid synthesis [31].

Methanogenesis is the main metabolic process in autotrophs from *Euryarchaeota*. Class I methanogens produce methane from CO_2 in a pathway called hydrogenotrophic. The electrons required for CO_2 reduction come from the oxidation of H_2 and are transferred to the carriers like ferredoxin and coenzyme F420 and ultimately to CO_2 in successive reactions [32].

In class II methanogens, besides the hydrogenotrophic pathway [33], two variants have also been found: acetoclastic and methylotrophic methanogenesis, both of which have a more recent evolutive origin [34]. In acetoclastic methanogenesis, one molecule of methane and one of CO_2 are generated from one molecule of acetate [35, 36]. Acetate is first converted to Acetyl-CoA by the action of the Acetyl-CoA synthetase enzyme with a concomitant expenditure of ATP. Later, the methyl group of Acetyl-CoA enters methanogenesis and gets reduced to generate methane in a process whose stages are shared with hydrogenotrophic methanogenesis. The electrons required to carry out the process are provided by the oxidation of the carbonyl group of Acetyl-CoA to carbon monoxide and then to CO_2 in a ferredoxin-dependent process.

In the methylotrophic methanogenesis, methane can be produced from the methyl group of several molecules, such as methanol, methylamine, and methanethiol. A total of four methyl groups are metabolized, and three of them enter methanogenesis where they are reduced to yield three methane molecules [35, 37]. The fourth methyl group is oxidized through a process equivalent to hydrogenotrophic methanogenesis, but it occurs in reverse order, yielding CO_2 and providing the electrons needed for the reduction of the other three molecules. The CO_2 produced in this process, as well as the one produced in acetoclastic methanogenesis, can enter in the reductive acetyl-CoA pathway to be destined to biomass generation.

4. Archaeal membrane lipids

Archaea are generally characterized by the unique structure of their membrane lipids. Their phospholipid composition mainly includes long chains of methylated isoprenoids attached to a glycerol-1-phosphate molecule via an ether bond, which has been suggested to contribute to the survival in extreme environments [38]. Archaeal lipids differ in isoprenoids chain length, composition, configuration, and various modifications at the polar head groups. The two main core structures are C_{20} sn-2, 3-diphytanyl glycerol diether lipid (also known as archaeal) and C_{40} sn-2, 3-diphytanyl diglyceroltetraether also known as glycerol diphytanoyl diglycerol tetraether (GDGT) or caldarchaeol. The archaeal lipids include some lipids with C_{25}isoprenoid chain, which enables the formation of the bilayer membrane. On the other hand, in caldarchaeol, two identical or different glycerol moieties are connected by two C_{40} isoprenoid chains, enabling the formation of monolayer membrane (**Figure 3**). These membranes present a higher degree of compactness compared to the other bilayer

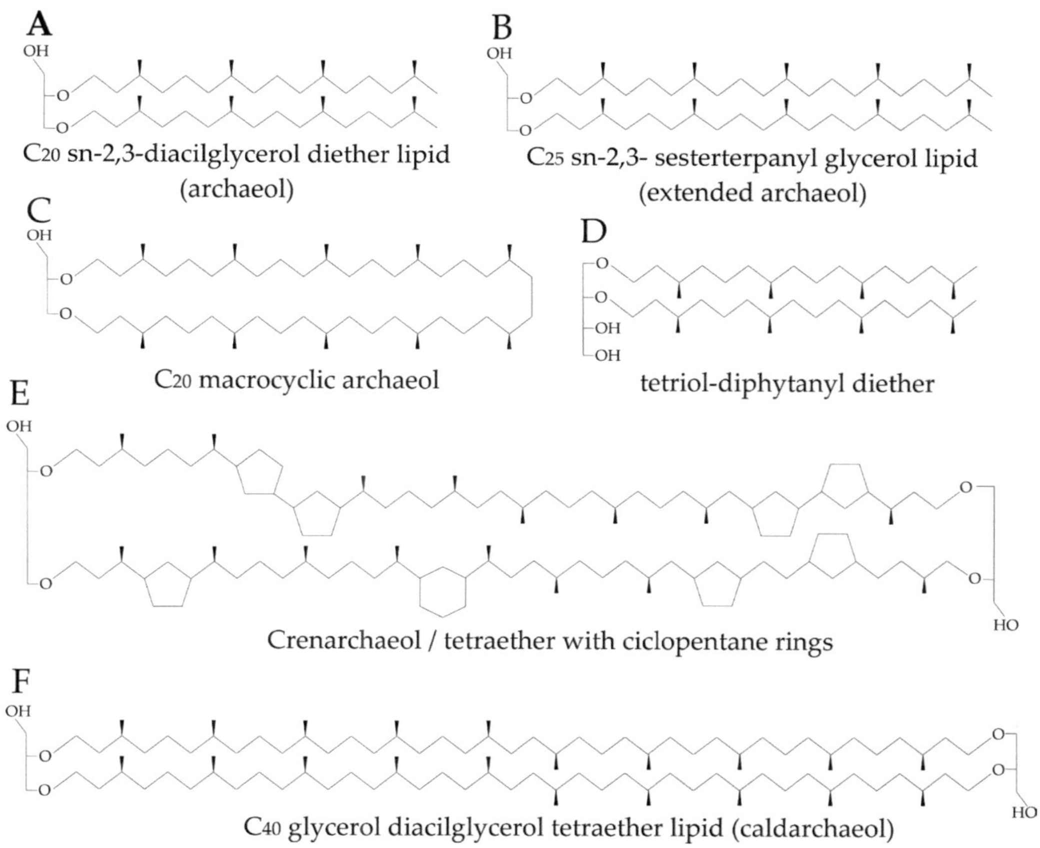

Figure 3. The structures of archaeal membrane lipids. (A) Archaeal C_{20}. (B) Modified archaeal C_{25}. (C) Macrocyclic archaeal. (D) Tetriol-archaeoldiether lipids. (E) Crenarchaeol with cyclopentane and cyclohexane. (F) Caldarchaeol C_{40} (GDGT).

membranes, which precludes external and internal layer fusion at high temperatures [39]. Furthermore, the ether bond typical of archaeal lipids is less susceptible to hydrolysis than the ester bonds present in bacterial lipids, which makes this kind of membrane to be more stable at high temperatures and in acidic environments. Molecular dynamic simulations have confirmed the importance of the monolayer structure in the membrane stability and determined that the presence of cyclic structures, like cyclopentane, increases membrane rigidity, rendering the membrane more resistant to mechanical stresses and high temperatures [40]. In hyperthermophilic archaea, the number of cyclic structures increases with the increase in growth temperature since the interaction between the lipids with cyclopentane is more stable. On the other hand, in psychrophilic *Euryarchaeota* the membrane lipids present unsaturated isoprenoid chains, which offer higher membrane fluidity at low temperatures. This is the case for the membranes from the psychrophilic organism *Methanococcoides burtonii,* where the identified lipids correspond to unsaturated archaeal lipids such as archaeal phosphatidylglycerol, archaeal phosphatidylinositol, hydroxyarchaeol phosphatidylglycerol, and hydroxyarchaeol phosphatidylinositol [41].

As a ubiquitous characteristic, the membrane lipids in *Halobacteria* organisms lack phospholipids with ethanolamine, inositol, and serine groups. Archaetidyl glycerol methyl phosphate (PGP-Me) is the main component of the membrane, which accounts for 50–80% of the total lipids. This particular lipid composition allows that the membranes from *Halobacteria* organisms retain their stability and impermeability in environments up to 4 M NaCl, distinct from the membranes of other *Euryarchaeota* organisms lacking PGP-Me [42].

Archaeal and extended archaeal are the main lipids in the orders *Methanococcales* and *Methanosarcinales,* while the orders *Methanopyrales, Thermoplasmatales, Archaeoglobales,* and *Methanomicrobiales* contain GDGTs lipids [39]. In the orders, *Thermococcales* and *Methanobacteriales,* both type of lipids, archaeal and GDGT, are present. Furthermore, in hyperthermophilic *Euryarchaeota* such as *Thermococcales* and *Thermoplasmatales,* GDGT with cyclic structures can be found (**Table 1**) [38, 43].

During the lipid synthesis in archaea, the isopentenyl diphosphate (IPP) and dimethyl allyl diphosphate (DMAPP) compounds serve as the building blocks of the isoprenoid chains. There are two pathways for the synthesis of these compounds: one of them corresponds to the mevalonate pathway (MVA), and the other is mevalonate-independent, which is known as C-methyl-D-erythritol-4-phosphate/1-deoxy-D-xylulose-5-phosphate (MEP-DOXP). In the MVA pathway, IPP and DMAPP are formed by the condensation of Acetyl-CoA molecules to give 3-hydroxy-3-methylglutaryl-CoA (HMG-CoA), which is later reduced to mevalonate and then phosphorylated and decarboxylated to form the precursor molecules of the isoprenoid chains [43]. Further, *M. jannaschii* uses a modified MVA pathway, where the conversion of mevalonate-5-phosphate to IP is catalyzed by a phosphomevalonate decarboxylase (MJ0403), and later IP is phosphorylated by the action of the IP kinase (MJ0044) enzyme [44].

Isoprenoid synthesis through the mevalonate-independent pathway was described initially in eukaryotes and later in bacteria, algae, and plants. Both pathways differ in the substrates and enzymes that participate in IPP formation. For example, in the MEP-DOXP pathway,

http://dx.doi.org/10.5772/intechopen.69943

Euryarchaeota order	Organism characteristic	Organism	Metabolism	Type of lipid	References
Halobacteriales	Psychrophilic Mesophilic	*Halobacterium* sp *Halorubrum lacusprofundi*	Heterotrophic	Archaeal C_{20}*, Archaeal extended C_{25}**, GDGT C_{40} and Archaeal unsaturated (psychrophilic organisms only)	[52, 53]
Methanosarcinales	Thermophilic Mesophilic Psychrophilic	*Methanosarcina* sp *Methanococcoides burtonii*	Autotrophic	Archaeal C_{20}*, GDGT C_{40} and Archaeal unsaturated (psychrophilic organisms only)	[41, 54, 55]
Methanopyrales	Hyperthermophilic	*Methanopyrus kandleri*	Autotrophic	Archaeal C_{20}* with cyclic ring (the degree of cyclization increase with the increase of the T°) and unsaturated Archaeal	[56]
Methanococcales	Hyperthermophilic	*Methanocaldococcus jannaschii*	Autotrophic	Archaeal C_{20} macrocyclic Archaeal***	[44]
Thermococcales	Thermophilic Hyperthermophilic	*Pyrococcus horikoshii* *Thermococcus* sp	Heterotrophic	Archaeal C_{20}*, Cardarchaeol derivatives and GDGT with up to two cyclic rings	[56]
Methanobacteriales	Mesophilic Thermophilic	*Methanobacterium thermoautotrophicus*	Autotrophic	Archaeal C_{20}* or Archaeal extended C_{25}** and GDGT-0	[39]
Archaeoglobales	Mesophilic Thermophilic	*Archaeoglobus Fulgidus*	Heterotrophic	Archaeal C_{20}*, **Archaeal extended C_{25}** and GDGT with zero to two cyclic rings	[57]
Thermoplasmatales	Mesophilic Thermophilic	*Thermoplasma acidophilum*	Heterotrophic	GDGT with one to three cyclic ring	[56]

Notes: *Archaeal C_{20} = C20 sn-2,3-diacilglycerol diether lipid.

**Archaeal C_{25} = C_{25} sn-2,3-sesterterpanyl.

***Macrocyclic Archaeal = C20 macrocyclic archaeal; GDGT = glycerol diphytanoyl glycerol tetraether; GDGT-0 cyclic ring; GDGT-1-4 cyclic ring; GDGT-5-8 cyclic ring.

Table 1. Main membrane lipids in *Euryarchaeota*.

the initial substrates for IPP formation are pyruvate and glyceraldehyde-3P, while in the MVA pathway are acetyl-CoA and acetoacetyl-CoA. Another difference lies in the last three enzymes of both pathways; in the MEP-DOXP route, they correspond to methylerythritol cyclodiphosphate (MEcPP) synthase and hydroxymethylbutenyl 4-diphosphate (HMBPP) synthase, which are absent in the MVA route. Further, the last enzyme in the MEP-DOXP pathway is an HMBPP reductase, which, in the other pathway, is a mevalonate-5-diphosphate (MVAPP) decarboxylase [45, 46].

5. Structural adaptations of extremophilic proteins

As already mentioned, archaea thrive in many different extremes: heat, cold, acid, base, salinity, pressure, and radiation. These harsh environmental conditions imposed several restrictions to which they had to adapt during the course of their evolution. Considering these extreme environments, archaea can be divided into: halophiles, psychrophiles, thermophiles, acidophiles, and piezophiles. However, it has to be remembered that these branches frequently intersect in interesting ways.

Archaeal organisms have evolved to deal with one or more extreme conditions that have led them to accumulate the changes mostly concerned with protein structure and enzyme activity. These adaptations made them a vast repertoire of macromolecules with particular features not available in their counterparts from other organisms. This constitutes an inexhaustible source of biological molecules for industrial or biotechnological applications.

5.1. Thermophiles and hyperthermophiles

Thermophilic and hyperthermophilic archaea are found mainly in the deep ocean, hydrothermal vents, and hot water near volcanoes. According to their growth temperature, these organisms have been classified as thermophiles or hyperthermophiles. The former are those able to grow at temperatures above 50°C and the latter at 80°C or more [47]. There are diverse cellular mechanisms that make the life possible at these extreme temperatures. The expression of molecular chaperones (HsP) that help in the correct folding of proteins and enzymes accompanied with more rigid membranes and proteins than those found in mesophiles are common characteristics of this kind of organisms [39, 48, 49]. At a genomic level, it is not clear if an increase in the G+C content is indeed a characteristic of thermophilic and hyperthermophilic organisms since some mesophilic organisms do show a higher proportion of these nitrogen bases than their hyperthermophilic counterparts [47, 50]. The high thermal stability, as well as the capacity of the enzymes of these microorganisms to catalyze reactions at very high temperatures, has made them a subject of intense research. Many archaeal thermophilic and hyperthermophilic enzymes employ substrates that are different from those used by their bacterial homologs; even some of them possess novel catalytic activities not found in bacteria, which make the archaeal enzymes a promising source for biotechnological processes.

Thermophilic and hyperthermophilic archaea could be either methanogenic or nonmethanogenic organisms. The nonmethanogenic hyperthermophilic archaea belong to the orders *Thermococcales*, *Thermoplasmatales*, and *Archaeoglobales*, whereas class I methanogenic archaea belong to the thermophilic organisms of the orders *Methanopyrales*, *Methanobacteriales*, and *Methanococcales* and class II methanogens belong to the orders *Methanomicrobiales* and *Methanosarcinales*.

5.1.1. Mechanism of protein adaptation to the heat

In general terms, the enzyme structures of thermophilic and hyperthermophilic archaea have been described as highly rigid and thermostable compared to their mesophilic homologs. The mechanisms reported to achieve this enhancement in thermostability include an increase in the number of ionic interactions, disulfide bridges, surface charges, higher oligomerization states, and a more compact hydrophobic core [51]. Although to date there are many characterized thermophilic and hyperthermophilic enzymes from the phylum *Euryarchaeota*, it is not possible to compare them with their mesophilic homologs from the same phylum due to the lack of studies regarding the homologous counterpart.

The structure of enzyme triose phosphate isomerase is characterized by TIM barrel fold, and it catalyzes the reversible interconversion of glyceraldehyde-3P and dihydroxyacetone phosphate. In eukaryotes, bacteria, and mesophilic archaea, this enzyme is a dimer, while in thermophilic and hyperthermophilic archaea, it exists in a tetrameric form [58]. The hyperthermophilic triose phosphate isomerase from *P. furiosus* and *Thermococcus onnurineus* was also characterized as tetramers [59]. The increase in the state of oligomerization could be a difference related to an increase in the thermal stability; an interesting but different example of oligomerization state as a strategy to increase thermostability is manifested by an amylase from *P. furiosus*. This hyperthermophilic enzyme, unlike its mesophilic homologs, which are dimers, presents a lower oligomerization state, being described as a highly packed monomer. This highly packed structure, as well as the decrease in the oligomerization state, results in the decrease in the hydrophobic surface exposed to the solvent [60]. In this case, the interactions that favor the compactness of the hydrophobic core of the hyperthermophilic amylase are hydrogen bonds, which play a fundamental role in maintaining the folding at high temperatures [60]. In order to analyze the importance of ionic and noncovalent interactions in the thermostability, Vogt et al. performed a comparative analysis between the mesophilic and thermophilic proteins employing 56 model proteins belonging to 16 families and concluded that in thermophilic proteins, interactions like hydrogen bonds are in a greater number than in mesophilic proteins, which are bestowed by a high number of charged residues constituting a key characteristic to increase thermostability [61]. In addition, it can be noted that thermophilic and hyperthermophilic proteins exhibit a larger polar surface exposed to the solvent in comparison with mesophilic proteins mainly due to the presence of charged residues on the surface and the diminution in the number of noncharged polar residues [62]. The presence of large hydrophobic lateral chains is also a characteristic of thermostable proteins. The comparison of the glutamate dehydrogenase from *P. furiosus* with its bacterial homologs (*Thermotoga marítima*, *Tm*GDH and *Clostridium symbiosum*, *Cs*GDH) shows that this thermostable enzyme presents a greater fraction of charged residues given mainly by arginine residues. In addition, it was established that the ionic-pair strategy follows this trend: *Pf*GDH > *Tm*GDH > *Cs*GDH [63].

A good example of the role of ionic interactions in the adaptation of protein structures to high temperatures is the ionic network present in a triose phosphate isomerase from *P. furiosus* and *T. onnurineus*; this type of ionic network is absent in the psychrophilic homolog from *Methanosarcinales* (*M. burtonii*) [64]. The introduction of ionic interactions in a psychrophilic enzyme significantly increased the thermal stability of a mutant, highlighting the importance of this type of interactions in the increased thermal stability of enzymes from archaea [64]. Even more, when this network of ionic interactions was eliminated from the triose phosphate isomerase from *P. furiosus*, its stability decreased [65].

An example of the use of disulfide bridges for increased stability is the comparison between the archaeal hyperthermophilic enzyme alpha-amylase from *P. furiosus* and its bacterial counterpart from *Bacillus licheniformis*. The study shows that the increased stability of the alpha-amylase from *P. furiosus* was due to a higher content of cysteine residues than the ones observed in the enzyme from *B. licheniformis*. The increase in cysteine residues along with the increase in the number of ionic pairs has been described as the main characteristics responsible for the activity and protein stabilization in this hyperthermophilic organism [66].

5.2. Psychrophiles

Most of the archaeal organisms studied evolved to colonize low-temperature aquatic ecosystems such as those present in Antarctic, Arctic, vast tracts of the deep sea, and also alpine regions. These organisms are called psychrophiles and can be classified in *Stenopsychrophiles* and *Eurypsychrophiles* according to their growth temperature range [67]. This classification is based on two parameters: optimal growth temperature (T_{opt}) and maximal growth temperature (T_{max}). *Stenopsychrophiles* show an upper optimal growth temperature less than ~20°C and a T_{max} not greater than 25°C. On the other hand, *Eurypsychrophiles* tolerate a broader temperature range, presenting T_{opt} above 30°C and T_{max} below 10°C [67]. To date, almost all psychrophilic archaea belong to the phylum *Euryarchaeota* and they are all methanogenic. Psychrophilic and methanogenic archaea can be found in the following archaeal orders: *Methanobacteriales, Methanomicrobiales,* and *Methanosarcinales*. *Methanobacterium* sp. is a representative of the order *Methanobacteriales,* while in the order *Methanomicrobiales,* we can find *Methanogenium frigidum, Methanogenium marinum,* and *Methanogenium boonei*. In *Methanosarcinales,* the organisms identified correspond to *M. burtonii, Methanococcoides alaskaense, Methanosarcina baltica, Methanosarcina lacustris,* and *Methanolobus psychrophilus*. Psychrophilic archaea and their proteins and enzymes have been a focus of great attention owing to their high potential as biocatalysts in biotechnological applications since a long time.

5.2.1. Mechanism of protein adaptation to the cold

Low temperature imposes several challenges to cellular functions such as replication, transcription, translation, and metabolic reactions crucial for the development of microorganisms. At a cellular level, the common strategies employed to cope low temperatures include, inter alia, cold shock proteins, antifreeze proteins, and an increased membrane fluidity [67]. Besides this, the protein structure should also adapt to a cold environment. Identifying the important features that confer specific thermal properties has been a subject of intense research in the last few years. Even so, to date, very few proteins from psychrophilic archaea have been studied, in contrast to a large number of proteins and enzymes from mesophilic, thermophilic, and hyperthermophilic archaea. The current studies indicate that the main feature of psychrophilic proteins and enzymes is to have a flexible structure, which could offset the energy decrease of the reaction medium, thus facilitating catalysis processes at low temperatures. Heat-induced unfolding experiments for psychrophilic, mesophilic, and thermophilic proteins show distinct stability patterns where the unfolding of the cold-adapted proteins occurs at lower temperatures (T_m) and gradually increases for the other groups [68]. Nonetheless, the psychrophilic enzymes do not display unusual or exotic 3D conformations and bear overall folds resembling that of their mesophilic counterparts [69]. The main challenge faced by psychrophilic enzymes is to catalyze reactions at an appropriate rate even when the low temperatures strongly diminish the rates of chemical reactions. Several reports regarding cold-active enzymes have demonstrated that they display a much higher specific activity at low and moderate temperatures as their thermophilic counterparts [70]. This is caused by the destabilization of either the active site or the whole protein, conferring mobility and flexibility to the active site at the temperatures that tend to freeze molecular motions [71]. It is generally accepted that although other molecular traits can contribute to cold activity, the lack of selective pressure on stable proteins, in conjunction with a strong selection of highly active enzymes, is the main factors responsible for cold activity adaptation in natural environments.

The psychrophilic enzymes from archaea evolved to attain more flexible structures by adopting several mechanisms. For example, by reducing the number of charged residues present at both the protein surface and the hydrophobic core (Arg, Lys, Glu). A low content of arginine residues results in a low number of hydrogen bonds that can be formed contributing to structural flexibility. In order to compensate for the loss of charges at the protein surface and avoid aggregation, these proteins present a great proportion of noncharged polar residues such as Gln and Thr, which in turn implies a decrease in stabilizing ion pairs favoring a structural destabilization [72]. Other adaptations include the clustering of glycine residues (providing local mobility), the disappearance of proline residues in loops (providing enhanced chain flexibility between secondary structures), as well as a lower number of ion pairs, aromatic interactions, and hydrogen bonds [73]. Additionally, the hydrophobicity of the protein core and the compactness of the protein interior is usually low [73]. In summary, all aforementioned factors are attenuated in strength and number in the structures of cold-active enzymes.

One remarkable fact about psychrophilic enzymes is that they are inactivated at the temperatures that are well below than the one at which the protein unfolds; this presents a remarkable difference from their mesophilic or thermophilic homologs. This led to the concept of a localized increase in the flexibility at the active site, which is responsible for a high but heat-labile activity, while the other regions of the protein, not involved in catalysis, might not have low stability [74, 75]. The comparison of the experimentally measured activation energy of transition ($\Delta G^{\neq}$) of some cold-active enzymes revealed that this parameter is systematically lower than the mesophilic proteins [74]. It has been proposed that the activation of these enzymes is facilitated by a decrease in the affinity of the enzyme for the substrate (higher level of ES) and by a possibly lower energetic level of $ES^{\neq}$. In many cases, the high activity of these enzymes at low temperatures has been associated with a rather open structure and also to a loss of specificity [73, 74].

The above and the other structural alterations have been reported mainly for psychrophilic enzymes from bacteria and eukarya, and there are not enough studies about psychrophilic archaeal enzymes in order to sustain that the same alternations are also responsible for cold adaptations in these organisms. A general adaptive mechanism proposed for psychrophilic enzymes from bacteria is the optimization of k_{cat} at the expense of K_m [73]. Although this mechanism is generally accepted, it cannot be generalized to archaeal enzymes considering the few cases studied. In the case of the GTPase of the elongation factor 2 (EF2) from *M. burtonii*, the adaptive mechanism to perform its activity at low temperatures involves a reduction in the K_m value compared to its thermophilic homolog phylogenetically related from *Methanosarcina thermophile* [76]. This decrease is due to the loss of noncovalent interactions that allow this enzyme to have a greater structural flexibility [76]. The loss of ionic and noncovalent interactions offering an increase in the structural flexibility has also been seen in other psychrophilic archaea enzymes such as the enzyme triphosphate isomerase from *M. burtonii* and in the DNA polymerase from *Cenarchaeum symbiosum* [77, 78].

The biophysical and catalytic features of psychrophilic enzymes present a challenge and offer an interesting model to unravel protein evolution, folding, and dynamics. We hope that these traits along with their tremendous biotechnological potentials will bring further promising advances in the archaeal psychrophilic protein research.

5.3. Halophiles

Hypersaline environments are defined as those containing higher salt concentrations than seawater (>3.5% total dissolved salts). Most hypersaline bodies are thalassohaline, dominated by Na^+, Ca^{2+}, Cl^-, and SO^{4-} ions, generally bearing neutral pH. These bodies derive from the evaporation of seawater and retain the relative proportion of salts in the sea. On the other hand, there is another less common group called athalassohaline of water bodies, dominated, among others, by Ca^{2+}, Mg^{2+}, Cl^-, and Ba^-, with pH conditions ranging from acidic to alkaline, and having a nonmarine origin. Both overall salinity and ionic composition together with the conditions like temperature and nutrient availability determine the existence of highly variable hypersaline environments that can be found extending from Antarctica to alkaline hypersaline soda brines and subterranean evaporite deposits.

Halophilic microorganisms are classically categorized according to their optimal growth at different salt concentrations, and two main groups have been recognized: the extreme halophiles (optimal growth above 15% NaCl) and moderate halophiles (optimal growth 3–15% NaCl).

In archaea, the only halophilic organisms known to date belong to the phylum *Euryarchaeota*. These organisms are distributed into three groups: (1) class *Halobacteria*, whose members are extreme halophiles that require over 3M salinity for growth and structural stability; (2) order *Methanosarcinales*, including extreme and moderate halophilic organisms; and (3) the recently discovered archaeal class, *Nanohaloarchaea*, uncultured to date [79, 80].

5.3.1. Mechanism of protein adaptation to salt

How do these organisms deal with high salinity environments and what adaptations did they incorporate into their molecular machinery and proteins? Both questions have been addressed in multiple studies with the main focus on *Halobacteria* organisms and their molecular machinery and proteins [51]. There are two fundamentally different strategies proposed for halophilic microorganisms explaining how they maintain osmotic pressure in their cytoplasm while growing in a saline medium: the salt-in-cytoplasm and the organic osmolyte accumulation. It has been demonstrated that, in *Halobacteria*, the intracellular accumulation of inorganic ions, mainly potassium and chloride, to high concentrations is the strategy employed to balance the extracellular osmotic pressure [81] in accordance with the salt-in mechanism. These high intracellular concentrations require unique adaptations of the molecular machinery implying that the proteins must retain their structural and functional integrity under such high salt conditions [80]. Although a perfect model that accurately explains how a protein structure is stabilized at high salt concentrations is still debatable, some specialized features of osmoadaptation have been identified through the determination of the genome sequence of *Halobacteria* organisms [82]. The statistical and bioinformatic analyses of these data, together with previous experimental data [83], have identified a biased amino acid composition known as the "halophilic signature." This signature is characterized by an increase in negative residues Asp and Glu, a reduction in the positively charged residues, Lys but no Arg, the low content of bulky hydrophobic residues like Phe and Ile, and an increase in small hydrophobic residues like Ala and Val [84]. As a result, in addition to preserving the protein folding relative to mesophilic counterparts, halophilic proteins exhibit a low hydrophobic content and a surface with a large negative net charge. This trend has also been confirmed by the means of isoelectric point calculated from the proteome of these organisms (the most acidic proteomes to date) [82].

The classical "solvation-stabilization" model proposed for the understanding of the mechanism behind the adaptation of the halophilic proteins proposes that the stability at high salt concentrations arises from the recruitment of an orderly solvate envelope of high ionic concentration, coordinated through the abundance of carboxylate groups (Asp and Glu) at the protein surface [85]. Despite the studies that have identified an increased stability and solubility of proteins enriched in Asp and Glu residues [86], biophysical [87] and crystallographic data [88] have failed to identify such hydration layers up to the extent proposed. More recently, it has been proposed that the main change in residue composition responsible for "halophilicity" is the diminution of Lys residues [89] due to the decreased solvent accessible area. This idea was confirmed by crystallographic studies, showing that water molecules adopt more structured distributions in the vicinity of Lys residues [90].

On the other hand, *Methanosarcinales* constitutes a heterogeneous group of organisms, consisting of the species with different salt requirements, ranging from moderate to extreme halophiles. These organisms are able to accumulate intracellular organic solutes, and the more halophilic organisms of the group are also able to accumulate inorganic ions (like K^+) in high concentrations [91]. Interestingly, recent phylogenetic studies show that this group of organisms branched off from the same ancestral node as the groups *Halobacteria* and *Nanohaloarchaea* [79]. Nevertheless, no study to date has addressed the possible adaptations on the amino acid composition and structural properties of proteins from *Methanosarcinales*.

5.4. Acidophiles

Acidophilic and acid tolerant organisms can thrive in natural, as well as man-made, acidic environments at pH less than 4.0. These environments are usually present in the combinations with other stressors, like high temperatures, elevated concentrations of heavy metals, and salinities approaching saturation [92]. As a result, *Euryarchaeota* acidophilic organisms are mostly polyextremophiles, being an example of acidophilic organisms that thrive in high salinities (*Halarchaeum* genera) [93] and in heavy metals along with high temperatures (*Thermoplasmata* class) [94].

Although some members of *Euryarchaeota* live in environments with pH values below 1, it has been demonstrated that most acidophiles maintain their internal pH close to neutrality. In order to adapt to these conditions, acidophilic organisms have evolved different mechanisms, such as a proton impermeable cell membrane, reversed membrane potential, and a cytoplasmic buffering system [95]. However, despite keeping their internal environment close to neutral pH values, these organisms possess macromolecules with adaptations that preserve their structure and function. However, the exact mechanisms underlying these adaptations have not been elucidated to date.

5.4.1. Mechanism of protein adaptation to acid

One striking feature of some acidophilic proteins is their requirement of a low pH (2–5) for their optimal activity, such as alfa-glucosidase and carboxyl esterase [96], even when the internal pH of these organisms is close to neutrality. Nevertheless, not all proteins from *Euryarchaeota* acidophiles have a preference for a low pH for their optimal activity, for example, an ATP-dependent DNA ligase from *Ferroplasma acidarmanus* has its optimal activity at pH 6–7, similar to the DNA ligases from nonacidophilic organisms [51, 97].

A possible explanation for the optimal activity at low pH was proposed through the study of the endo-β-glucanase from the *Crenarchaeota Sulfolobus solfataricus* [98]. This enzyme has an optimum pH of approximately 2.0 and an optimum temperature around 80°C. Through homology modeling, it was determined that its catalytic domain possesses a fold similar to that observed in other mesophilic, acidophilic, and neutral cellulases and its surface displays mostly negative charges. Nonetheless, other β-glucanases from mesophilic homologs, which are optimally active at neutral pH, also display low predicted P.I. values, which suggests that the net charge is not the only factor responsible for the extreme acidic stability [51, 98].

Recent crystallographic studies shed some light on the mechanisms of protein stability and catalytic efficiency at low pH. The strategy of increased negative residues was not present at the same extent in the aspartate racemase from *P. torridus* [99], while in the carboxylesterase from *F. acidiphilum* a highly negatively charged surface around the active site was identified. However, this is not a trend observed for the rest of the protein surface. Further, in this enzyme, it has been demonstrated that the modifications in the hydrogen bond network surrounding the catalytic triad altered the catalytic efficiency and allowed pH preference adjustments from a low pH to a more upward optimum and vice versa [100].

5.5. Piezophiles

Deep-sea hydrothermal vents are another extreme environment colonized by archaea. In these environments, an average pressure of approximately 38 MPa is found that can reach

http://dx.doi.org/10.5772/intechopen.69943

even up to 110 MPa, hence imposing a major challenge for life. Organisms that can thrive in such extreme barometric pressure are often termed as piezophiles or barophiles. Several piezophiles have been cultured; however, they require specialized equipment in order to maintain high pressures. Thus, many studies have focused on nonculturing techniques, like genomic analysis. Besides high pressure, hydrothermal vents also have very high temperatures and indeed could be the habitat of hyperthermophiles. However, only a few hyperthermophiles are also piezophiles. To date, the only strictly piezophilic anaerobic hyperthermophilic archaeon reported is *Pyrococcus yayanosii* CH1 [101]. Some reports have indicated that there are no specific pressure-related adaptations required for the enzymes isolated from piezophiles to be stable; however, a hydrostatic pressure asymmetry index (PAI) that reflects the extent to which an amino acid is preferred by piezophiles has been described [102]. Proteomic comparative analysis of *P. furiosus* and *P. abyssi* shows that Asp and Arg are the only two amino acids that can be designated preferentially barophilic, although previous studies designated five (Arg, Ser, Val, Asp, and Gly). On the other hand, only three amino acids (Asn, Lys, and Thr) display a clear preference for nonbarophily [103].

6. Biotechnological applications of extremozymes

The extreme harsh environmental conditions where extremophiles live serve as an enormous source of enzymes with peculiar properties that make them very suitable for industrial or biotechnological applications. The first commercialized enzyme was diastase, available in the market since 1830 in France. Since then, the enzyme market gained importance because they not only reduce the cost of the products but benefit the environment. In 2015, the global market for industrial enzymes reached nearly 4.9 billion and is expected to reach nearly $5.0 billion in 2016 to $6.3 billion in 2021. Food and animal feed industrial enzyme market is expected to grow to $1.9 billion and $1.6 billion in 2021, respectively (BCC Research Biotechnology report 2017). At present, most of the industrially applied enzymes show low activity and stability, which is highly disadvantageous in terms of concomitant high costs (**Table 2**).

There have been continuous efforts for expressing the genes encoding for the enzymes from extremophiles in mesophilic hosts in order to overproduce them and modify their properties to be suitable for commercial applications. In addition, archaeal enzyme expression can be achieved by using extremophilic microorganisms as hosts for autologous gene expression [124]. Integrative and shuttle vectors have been developed for *Methanococcus* species, which allow overexpressing specific enzymes with complex prosthetic groups that are inactive if expressed in *E. coli* [124].

Archaeal compounds also have many applications in the pharmaceutical and alimentary industry. *Haloarchaea* organisms from the order *Halobacterium* (*Haloferax* sp.) produce a peptide called halocin, which is used as an antimicrobial and preservative in food with high salt content. For example, the H6/H7 halocin produced by *Haloferax gibbonsii* affects the Na+/H+ antiporter and then inhibits the membrane ionic gradient of the target cell, provoking cell death by lysis [125, 126]. In addition, compounds like canthaxanthin produced by *Haloferax*

Enzyme	Enzyme characteristics	Organism	Application	References
α-Amylase	Hyperthermophilic	*Thermococcus profundus*	Bread and baking industry, Starch liquefaction and saccharification. Production of glucose, fructose for sweeteners, textile desizing, paper industry	[104]
	Halophilic	*Haloferax mediterranei*		[105]
	Acidophilic	*Picrophilus torridus*		Q6KZM7*
	Psychrophilic	*Methanococcoides burtonii*		Q12YQ1*
Subtilisin	Hyperthermophilic	*Thermococcus kodakaraensis*	Detergents, baking, brewing and amino acid production	[106]
	Halophilic	*Halorubrum litoreum*		M0NQ93*
	Acidophilic	*Thermoplasmatales archaeon*		M7TYK7*
	Psychrophilic	*Methanolobus psychrophilus*		K4M7H8*
Esterase	Hyperthermophilic	*Picrophilus torridus*	Detergent formulations and dairy industry	[107]
	Halophilic	*Haloarcula marismortui*		[108]
	Acidophilic	*Picrophilus torridus*		[107]
DNA polymerase	Hyperthermophilic	*Pyrococcus abyssi*	DNA cloning, sequencing, labeling, mutagenesis, and other purposes	[109]
	Halophilic	*Halobacterium halobium*		[110]
	Acidophilic	*Thermoplasma acidophilum*		Q9HJR0*
	Psychrophilic	*Methanococcoides burtonii*		Q12YC5*
Cellulase	Hyperthermophilic	*Pyrococcus horikoshii*	Pulp and paper, textile, laundry, biofuel production	[111]
	Halophilic	*Halorhabdus utahensis*		[112]
	Acidophilic	*Picrophilus torridus*		Q6KZ15*
	Psychrophilic	*Methanococcoides burtonii*		Q12XZ9*
β-Glycosidase	Hyperthermophilic	*Pyrococcus furiosus*	Polymer degradation, color brightening, color extraction of juice, cotton products, synthesis of sugars	[113]
	Halophilic	*Haloarcula marismortui*		Q5V5G3*
	Acidophilic	*Picrophilus torridus*		[114]
β-Galactosidase	Hyperthermophilic	*Pyrococcus woesei*	Detergent and food industries and for the production of fine chemicals	[115]
	Halophilic	*Haloferax alicante*		[116]
	Acidophilic	*Picrophilus torridus*		[117]
	Psychrophilic	*Halorubrum lacusprofundi*		[118]

http://dx.doi.org/10.5772/intechopen.69943

Enzyme	Enzyme characteristics	Organism	Application	References
Alcohol dehydrogenase	Hyperthermophilic	*Thermococcus hydrothermalis*	Food, pharmaceutical, and fine chemicals industries	[119]
	Halophilic	*Haloferax volcanii*		[120]
	Acidophilic	*Thermoplasma acidophilum*		[121]
	Psychrophilic	*Halorubrum lacusprofundi*		B9LV78*
Lipase	Hyperthermophilic	*Pyrococcus furiosus*	Detergent formulations and the dairy industry	[122]
	Halophilic	*Natronococcus* sp		[123]
	Acidophilic	*Thermoplasma acidophilum*		Q9HJS7*

*UniProt code.

Table 2. Extremozymes and their applications in industrial and biotechnological processes.

alexandrinus present antioxidant properties that can be used potentially as food supplements to prevent cancer or cardiovascular diseases [127]. Other compounds like exopolysaccharides produced by *Haloferax* have been employed in the food industry as emulsifiers since they are stable at high temperatures. Other interesting biotechnological applications are the use of archaeal lipids for the formation of a new generation of liposomes, known as archaeosomes. Archaeal lipids present a more polar character and have ether bonds which gave them more stability at extreme temperatures, pH, and pressure. In addition, these characteristics provide protection against oxidation, to the action of phospholipases and chemical hydrolysis, providing an advantage over liposomes formed by neutral phospholipids. Owing to their great stability, biocompatibility, and biodegradation, archaeosomes have many uses as vaccine adjuvants and in drug delivery system [128].

There is a huge amount of information available regarding biotechnological applications of extremozymes, and therefore, this chapter made an effort to summarize the applications of these enzymes and compounds in some selected areas. Considering that very few archaeal enzymes have found their way to the market in some applications, we provided the examples of such extremophiles and the corresponding UniProt code for the homologous enzymes present in archaea (**Table 2**). We hope that this kind of information will be extremely valuable for future studies looking for archaeal enzymes with particular properties.

Acknowledgements

We would like to thank CONICYT for financial support: Fondecyt Postdoctorado N°3160332 to VC-F, Fondecyt Postdoctorado N°3160376 to AH-M, and Fondecyt Regular N°1150460 to VG.

Author details

Victor Castro-Fernandez*, Ricardo Zamora, Alejandra Herrera-Morande, Gabriel Vallejos, Felipe Gonzalez-Ordenes and Victoria Guixé*

*Address all correspondence to: vguixe@uchile.cl and vcasfe@ug.uchile.cl

Department of Biology, Faculty of Sciences, University of Chile, Santiago, Chile

References

[1] Huber R, Huber H, Stetter KO. Towards the ecology of hyperthermophiles: Biotopes, new isolation strategies and novel metabolic properties. FEMS Microbiology Reviews. 2000;**24**(5):615-623

[2] Cavicchioli R. Archaea—timeline of the third domain. Nature Reviews Microbiology. 2011;**9**(1):51-61

[3] Woese CR, Kandler O, Wheelis ML. Towards a natural system of organisms: Proposal for the domains Archaea, Bacteria, and Eucarya. Proceedings of the National Academy of Sciences of the United States of America. 1990;**87**(12):4576-4579

[4] Philippe H, Germot A. Phylogeny of eukaryotes based on ribosomal RNA: Long-branch attraction and models of sequence evolution. Molecular Biology and Evolution. 2000;**17**:830-834

[5] Pace NR. Mapping the tree of life: Progress and prospects. Microbiology and Molecular Biology Reviews. 2009;**73**(4):565-576

[6] Petitjean C, Deschamps P, López-García P, Moreira D, Brochier-Armanet C. Extending the conserved phylogenetic core of archaea disentangles the evolution of the third domain of life. Molecular Biology and Evolution. 2015;**32**(5):1242-1254

[7] Battistuzzia FU, Hedgesa SB. Archaebacteria. In: Hedges SB, Kumar S, editors. The Timetree of Life. New York: Oxford University Press; 2009. pp. 101-105

[8] Thorgersen MP, Stirrett K, Scott RA, Adams MWW. Mechanism of oxygen detoxification by the surprisingly oxygen-tolerant hyperthermophilic archaeon, *Pyrococcus furiosus*. Proceedings of the National Academy of Sciences of the United States of America. 2012;**109**(45):18547-18552

[9] Schönheit P, Buckel W, Martin WF. On the origin of heterotrophy. Trends in Microbiology. 2016;**24**(1):12-25

[10] Selkov E, Maltsev N, Olsen GJ, Overbeek R, Whitman WB. A reconstruction of the metabolism of *Methanococcus jannaschii* from sequence data. Gene. 1997;**197**(1-2):11-26

[11] Goyal N, Zhou Z, Karimi IA. Metabolic processes of *Methanococcus maripaludis* and potential applications. Microbial Cell Factories. 2016;**15**(1):107

[12] Santiago-Martínez MG, Encalada R, Lira-Silva E, Pineda E, Gallardo-Pérez JC, Reyes-García MA, et al. The nutritional status of *Methanosarcina acetivorans* regulates glycogen metabolism and gluconeogenesis and glycolysis fluxes. FEBS Journal. 2016;**283**(10):1979-1999

[13] Lee H, Shockley KR, Schut GJ, Conners SB, Montero CI, Matthew R, et al. Transcriptional and biochemical analysis of starch metabolism in the hyperthermophilic archaeon *Pyrococcus furiosus*. Journal of Bacteriology. 2006;**188**(6):2115-2125

[14] Schut GJ, Brehm SD, Datta S, Adams WW, Adams MWW. Whole-genome DNA microarray analysis of a hyperthermophile and an archaeon: *Pyrococcus furiosus* grown on carbohydrates or peptides. Journal of Bacteriology. 2003;**185**(13):3935-3947

[15] Vanfossen AL, Lewis DL, Nichols JD, Kelly RM. Polysaccharide degradation and synthesis by extremely thermophilic anaerobes. Annals of the New York Academy of Sciences. 2008;**1125**:322-337

[16] Bräsen C, Esser D, Rauch B, Siebers B. Carbohydrate metabolism in archaea: Current insights into unusual enzymes and pathways and their regulation. Microbiology and Molecular Biology Reviews. 2014;**78**(1):89-175

[17] Guixé V, Merino F. The ADP-dependent sugar kinase family: Kinetic and evolutionary aspects. IUBMB Life. 2009;**61**(7):753-761

[18] Currie MA, Merino F, Skarina T, Wong AHY, Singer A, Brown G, et al. ADP-dependent 6-phosphofructokinase from *Pyrococcus horikoshii* OT3: Structure determination and biochemical characterization of PH1645. Journal of Biological Chemistry. 2009;**284**(34):22664-22671

[19] Mukund S, Adams MWW. Glyceraldehyde-3-phosphate ferredoxin oxidoreductase, a novel tungsten-containing enzyme with a potential glycolytic role in the hyperthermophilic archaeon *Pyrococcus furiosus*. Journal of Biological Chemistry. 1995;**270**:8389-8392

[20] Ma K, Hutchins A, Sung SJ, Adams MW. Pyruvate ferredoxin oxidoreductase from the hyperthermophilic archaeon, *Pyrococcus furiosus*, functions as a CoA-dependent pyruvate decarboxylase. Proceedings of the National Academy of Sciences of the United States of America. 1997;**94**(18):9608-9613

[21] Sapra R, Bagramyan K, Adams MWW. A simple energy-conserving system: Proton reduction coupled to proton translocation. Proceedings of the National Academy of Sciences of the United States of America. 2003;**100**(13):7545-7550

[22] Schäfer T, Selig M, Schnheit P. Acetyl-CoA synthetase (ADP forming) in archaea, a novel enzyme involved in acetate formation and ATP synthesis. Archives of Microbiology. 1993;**159**:72-83

[23] Huynen MA, Dandekar T, Bork P. Variation and evolution of the citric-acid cycle: A genomic perspective. Trends in Microbiology. 1999;**7**(7):281-291

[24] Schut GJ, Bridger SL, Adams MWW. Insights into the metabolism of elemental sulfur by the hyperthermophilic archaeon *Pyrococcus furiosus*: Characterization of a coenzyme A-dependent NAD(P)H sulfur oxidoreductase. Journal of Bacteriology. 2007;**189**(12):4431-4441

[25] Sakuraba H, Yoshioka I, Koga S, Takahashi M, Kitahama Y, Satomura T, et al. ADP-dependent glucokinase/phosphofructokinase, a novel bifunctional enzyme from the hyperthermophilic archaeon *Methanococcus jannaschii*. Journal of Biological Chemistry. 2002;**277**(15):12495-12498

[26] Castro-Fernandez V, Bravo-Moraga F, Herrera-Morande A, Guixe V. Bifunctional ADP-dependent phosphofructokinase/glucokinase activity in the order *Methanococcales*—biochemical characterization of the mesophilic enzyme from *Methanococcus maripaludis*. FEBS Journal. 2014;**281**(8):2017-2029

[27] Yu JP, Ladapo J, Whitman WB. Pathway of glycogen metabolism in *Methanococcus maripaludis*. Journal of Bacteriology. 1994;**176**(2):325-332

[28] Hendrickson EL, Kaul R, Zhou Y, Bovee D, Chapman P, Chung J, et al. Complete genome sequence of the genetically tractable hydrogenotrophic methanogen *Methanococcus maripaludis*. Journal of Bacteriology. 2004;**186**(20):6956-6969

[29] Berg IA, Kockelkorn D, Ramos-Vera WH, Say RF, Zarzycki J, Hügler M, et al. Autotrophic carbon fixation in archaea. Nature Reviews Microbiology. 2010;**8**(6):447-460

[30] Hendrickson EL, Leigh JA. Roles of coenzyme F420-reducing hydrogenases and hydrogen- and F420-dependent methylenetetrahydromethanopterin dehydrogenases in reduction of F420 and production of hydrogen during methanogenesis. Journal of Bacteriology. 2008;**190**(14):4818-4821

[31] Furdui C, Ragsdale SW. The role of pyruvate ferredoxin oxidoreductase in pyruvate synthesis during autotrophic growth by the Wood-Ljungdahl pathway. Journal of Biological Chemistry. 2000;**275**(37):28494-28499

[32] Thauer RK. The Wolfe cycle comes full circle. Proceedings of the National Academy of Sciences of the United States of America. 2012;**109**(38):15084-15085

[33] Lessner DJ, Li L, Li Q, Rejtar T, Andreev VP, Reichlen M, et al. An unconventional pathway for reduction of CO_2 to methane in CO-grown *Methanosarcina acetivorans* revealed by proteomics. Proceedings of the National Academy of Sciences of the United States of America. 2006;**103**(47):17921-17926

[34] Fournier GP, Gogarten JP. Evolution of acetoclastic methanogenesis in *Methanosarcina* via horizontal gene transfer from cellulolytic Clostridia. Journal of Bacteriology. 2008;**190**(3):1124-1127

[35] Costa KC, Leigh JA. Metabolic versatility in methanogens. Current Opinion in Biotechnology. 2014;**29**(1):70-75

[36] Welte C, Deppenmeier U. Bioenergetics and anaerobic respiratory chains of aceticlastic methanogens. Biochimica et Biophysica Acta. 2014;**1837**(7):1130-1147

[37] Lieber DJ, Catlett J, Madayiputhiya N, Nandakumar R, Lopez MM, Metcalf WW, et al. A multienzyme complex channels substrates and electrons through acetyl-CoA and methane biosynthesis pathways in *Methanosarcina*. PLoS One. 2014;**9**(9):1-8

[38] Caforio A, Driessen AJM. Archaeal phospholipids: Structural properties and biosynthesis. Biochimica et Biophysica Acta. Doi:10.1016/j.bbalip.2016.12.006. [Epub ahead of print]

[39] Koga Y. Thermal adaptation of the archaeal and bacterial lipid membranes. Archaea. 2012;**2012**:789652. Doi:10.1016/j.bbalip.2016.12.006 [Epub]

[40] Shinoda W, Shinoda K, Baba T, Mikami M. Molecular dynamics study of bipolar tetraether lipid membranes. Biophysical Journal. 2005;**89**(5):3195-3202

[41] Nichols DS, Miller MR, Davies NW, Goodchild A, Raftery M, Cavicchioli R. Cold adaptation in the Antarctic archaeon *Methanococcoides burtonii* involves membrane lipid unsaturation. Journal of Bacteriology. 2004;**186**(24):8508-8515

[42] Tenchov B, Vescio EM, Sprott GD, Zeidel ML, Mathai JC. Salt tolerance of archaeal extremely halophilic lipid membranes. Journal of Biological Chemistry. 2006;**281**(15):10016-10023

[43] Villanueva L, Damsté JSS, Schouten S. A re-evaluation of the archaeal membrane lipid biosynthetic pathway. Nature Reviews Microbiology. 2014;**12**(6):438-448

[44] Grochowski LL, Xu H, White RH. *Methanocaldococcus jannaschii* uses a modified mevalonate pathway for biosynthesis of isopentenyl diphosphate. Journal of Bacteriology. 2006;**188**(9):3192-3198

[45] Coppens I. Targeting lipid biosynthesis and salvage in apicomplexan parasites for improved chemotherapies. Nature Reviews Microbiology. 2013;**11**(12):823-835

[46] Hunter WN. The non-mevalonate pathway of isoprenoid precursor biosynthesis. Journal of Biological Chemistry. 2007;**282**(30):21573-21577

[47] Urbieta MS, Donati ER, Chan KG, Shahar S, Sin LL, Goh KM. Thermophiles in the genomic era: Biodiversity, science, and applications. Biotechnology Advances. 2015;**33**(6):633-647

[48] Albers S-V, van de Vossenberg J, Driessen AJM, Konings W. Adaptations of the archaeal cell membrane to heat stress. Frontiers in Bioscience. 2000;**5**:813-820

[49] Haslbeck M, Kastenmüller A, Buchner J, Weinkauf S, Braun N. Structural dynamics of archaeal small heat shock proteins. Journal of Molecular Biology. 2008;**378**(2):362-374

[50] Hickey DA, Singer GAC. Genomic and proteomic adaptations to growth at high temperature. Genome Biology. 2004;**5**(10):117

[51] Reed CJ, Lewis H, Trejo E, Winston V, Evilia C. Protein adaptations in archaeal extremophiles. Archaea. 2013;**2013**

[52] Kamekura M, Kates M. Structural diversity of membrane lipids in members of *Halobacteriaceae*. Bioscience, Biotechnology, and Biochemistry. 1999;**63**(6):969-972

[53] Gibson JAE, Miller MR, Davies NW, Neill GP, Nichols DS, Volkman JK. Unsaturated diether lipids in the psychrotrophic archaeon *Halorubrum lacusprofundi*. Systematic and Applied Microbiology. 2005;**28**(1):19-26

[54] Sprott GD, Ekiel I, Patel GB. Metabolic pathways in *Methanococcus jannaschii* and other methanogenic bacteria. Applied and Environmental Microbiology. 1993;**59**(4):1092-1098

[55] Sprott GD, Agnew BJ, Patel GB. Structural features of ether lipids in the archaeobacterial thermophiles *Pyrococcus furiosus, Methanopyrus kandleri, Methanothermus fervidus,* and *Sulfolobus acidocaldarius*. Canadian Journal of Microbiology. 1997;**43**(5):467-476

[56] Oger PM, Cario A. Adaptation of the membrane in archaea. Biophysical Chemistry. 2013;**183**:42-56

[57] Lai D, Springstead JR, Monbouquette HG. Effect of growth temperature on ether lipid biochemistry in *Archaeoglobus fulgidus*. Extremophiles. 2008;**12**(2):271-278

[58] Walden H, Taylor GL, Lorentzen E, Pohl E, Lilie H, Schramm A, et al. Structure and function of a regulated archaeal triosephosphate isomerase adapted to high temperature. Journal of Molecular Biology. 2004;**342**(3):861-875

[59] Sharma P, Guptasarma P. "Super-perfect" enzymes: Structural stabilities and activities of recombinant triose phosphate isomerases from *Pyrococcus furiosus* and *Thermococcus onnurineus* produced in *Escherichia coli*. Biochemical and Biophysical Research Communications. 2015;**460**(3):753-758

[60] Park JT, Song HN, Jung TY, Lee MH, Park SG, Woo EJ, et al. A novel domain arrangement in a monomeric cyclodextrin-hydrolyzing enzyme from the hyperthermophile *Pyrococcus furiosus*. Biochimica et Biophysica Acta. 2013;**1834**(1):380-386

[61] Vogt G, Woell S, Argos P. Protein thermal stability, hydrogen bonds, and ion pairs. Journal of Molecular Biology. 1997;**269**(4):631-643

[62] Lee CF, Makhatadze GI, Wong KB. Effects of charge-to-alanine substitutions on the stability of ribosomal protein L30e from *Thermococcus celer*. Biochemistry. 2005;**44**(51):16817-16825

[63] Scandurra R, Consalvi V, Chiaraluce R, Politi L, Engel PC. Protein stability in extremophilic archaea. Frontiers in Bioscience. 2000;**5**:D787-D795

[64] Dhaunta N, Arora K, Chandrayan SK, Guptasarma P. Introduction of a thermophile-sourced ion pair network in the fourth beta/alpha unit of a psychophile-derived triosephosphate isomerase from *Methanococcoides burtonii* significantly increases its kinetic thermal stability. Biochimica et Biophysica Acta. 2013;**1834**(6):1023-1033

[65] Chandrayan SK, Guptasarma P. Attenuation of ionic interactions profoundly lowers the kinetic thermal stability of *Pyrococcus furiosus* triosephosphate isomerase. Biochimica et Biophysica Acta. 2009;**1794**(6):905-912

[66] Savchenko A, Vieille C, Kang S, Zeikus JG. *Pyrococcus furiosus* alpha-amylase is stabilized by calcium and zinc. Biochemistry. 2002;**41**(19):6193-6201

[67] Feller G, Gerday C. Psychrophilic enzymes: Hot topics in cold adaptation. Nature Reviews Microbiology. 2003;**1**(3):200-208

[68] Cipolla A, Delbrassine F, Da Lage JL, Feller G. Temperature adaptations in psychrophilic, mesophilic and thermophilic chloride-dependent alpha-amylases. Biochimie. 2012;**94**(9):1943-1950

[69] Somero GN. Adaptation of enzymes to temperature: Searching for basic "strategies." Comparative Biochemistry and Physiology. 2004;**139**(3):321-333

[70] Thomas T, Cavicchioli R. Effect of temperature on stability and activity of elongation factor 2 proteins from Antarctic and thermophilic methanogens. Journal of Bacteriology. 2000;**182**(5):1328-1332

[71] Fields PA, Somero GN. Hot spots in cold adaptation: Localized increases in conformational flexibility in lactate dehydrogenase A4 orthologs of Antarctic notothenioid fishes. Physiology. 1998;**95**(9):11476-11481

[72] Saunders NFW, Thomas T, Curmi PMG, Mattick JS, Kuczek E, Slade R, et al. Mechanisms of thermal adaptation revealed from the genomes of the Antarctic archaea *Methanogenium frigidum* and *Methanococcoides burtonii*. Genome Research. 2003;**13**(7):1580-1588

[73] Siddiqui KS, Cavicchioli R. Cold-adapted enzymes. Annual Review of Biochemistry. 2006;**75**:403-433

[74] Lonhienne T, Gerday C, Feller G. Psychrophilic enzymes: Revisiting the thermodynamic parameters of activation may explain local flexibility. Biochimica et Biophysica Acta. 2000;**1543**(1):1-10

[75] Chiuri R, Maiorano G, Rizzello A, Del Mercato LL, Cingolani R, Rinaldi R, et al. Exploring local flexibility/rigidity in psychrophilic and mesophilic carbonic anhydrases. Biophysical Journal. 2009;**96**(4):1586-1596

[76] Siddiqui KS, Cavicchioli R, Thomas T. Thermodynamic activation properties of elongation factor 2 (EF-2) proteins from psychrotolerant and thermophilic archaea. Extremophiles. 2002;**6**(2):143-150

[77] Uemori T, Ishino Y, Doi H, Kato I. The hyperthermophilic archaeon *Pyrodictium occultum* has two alpha-like DNA polymerases. Journal of Bacteriology. 1995;**177**(8):2164-2177

[78] Schleper C, Swanson RV, Mathur EJ. Characterization of a DNA polymerase from the uncultivated psychrophilic archaeon *Cenarchaeum symbiosum*. Journal of Bacteriology. 1997;**179**(24):7803-7811

[79] Narasingarao P, Podell S, Ugalde JA, Brochier-Armanet C, Emerson JB, Brocks JJ, et al. *De novo* metagenomic assembly reveals abundant novel major lineage of archaea in hypersaline microbial communities. ISME Journal. 2012;**6**(1):81-93

[80] Oren A. Microbial life at high salt concentrations: Phylogenetic and metabolic diversity. Saline Systems. 2008;**4**:2

[81] Christian JH, Waltho JA. Solute concentrations within cells of halophilic and non-halophilic bacteria. Biochimica et Biophysica Acta. 1962;**65**:506-508

[82] Kennedy SP, Ng WV, Salzberg SL, Hood L, DasSarma S. Understanding the adaptation of *Halobacterium* species NRC-1 to its extreme environment through computational analysis of its genome sequence. Genome Research. 2001;**11**(10):1641-1650

[83] Lanyi JK. Salt-dependent properties of proteins from extremely halophilic bacteria. Bacteriological Reviews. 1974;**38**(3):272-290

[84] Kastritis PL, Papandreou NC, Hamodrakas SJ. Haloadaptation: Insights from comparative modeling studies of halophilic archaeal DHFRs. International Journal of Biological Macromolecules. 2007;**41**(4):447-453

[85] Madern D, Ebel C, Zaccai G. Halophilic adaptation of enzymes. Extremophiles. 2000; **4**(2):91-99

[86] Kramer RM, Shende VR, Motl N, Pace CN, Scholtz JM. Toward a molecular understanding of protein solubility: Increased negative surface charge correlates with increased solubility. Biophysical Journal. 2012;**102**(8):1907-1915

[87] Qvist J, Ortega G, Tadeo X, Millet O, Halle B. Hydration dynamics of a halophilic protein in folded and unfolded states. Journal of Physical Chemistry B. 2012;**116**(10):3436-3444

[88] Britton KL, Baker PJ, Fisher M, Ruzheinikov S, Gilmour DJ, Bonete M-J, et al. Analysis of protein solvent interactions in glucose dehydrogenase from the extreme halophile *Haloferax mediterranei*. Proceedings of the National Academy of Sciences of the United States of America. 2006;**103**(13):4846-4851

[89] Tadeo X, López-Méndez B, Trigueros T, Laín A, Castaño D, Millet O. Structural basis for the amino acid composition of proteins from halophilic archaea. PLoS Biology. 2009;**7**(12):1-9

[90] Talon R, Coquelle N, Madern D, Girard E. An experimental point of view on hydration/solvation in halophilic proteins. Frontiers in Microbiology. 2014;**5**(2):1-8

[91] Lai MC, Gunsalus RP. Glycine betaine and potassium ion are the major compatible solutes in the extremely halophilic methanogen *Methanohalophilus strain* Z7302. Journal of Bacteriology. 1992;**174**(22):7474-7477

[92] Spijkerman E, Weithoff G. Acidic environments. In: Bell EM, editor. Life at Extremes: Environments, Organism and Strategies for Survival. Oxfordshire, UK: CABI; 2012. pp. 364-375

[93] Shimane Y, Minegishi H, Echigo A, Kamekura M, Itoh T, Ohkuma M, et al. *Halarchaeum grantii sp*. Nov., a moderately acidophilic haloarchaeon isolated from a commercial salt sample. International Journal of Systematic and Evolutionary Microbiology. 2015;**65**(11):3830-3835

[94] Huber, H., Stetter, K.O. *Thermoplasmatales*. In: The Prokaryotes. 3rd ed. New York: Springer; 2006. p.101-112

[95] Baker-Austin C, Dopson M. Life in acid: pH homeostasis in acidophiles. Trends in Microbiology. 2007;**15**(4):165-171

[96] Golyshina OV, Timmis KN. Ferroplasma and relatives, recently discovered cell wall-lacking archaea making a living in extremely acid, heavy metal-rich environments. Environmental Microbiology. 2005;**7**(9):1277-1288

[97] Jackson BR, Noble C, Lavesa-Curto M, Bond PL, Bowater RP. Characterization of an ATP-dependent DNA ligase from the acidophilic archaeon "*Ferroplasma acidarmanus*" Fer1. Extremophiles. 2007;**11**(2):315-327

[98] Huang Y, Krauss G, Cottaz S, Driguez H, Lipps G. A highly acid-stable and thermostable endo-beta-glucanase from the thermoacidophilic archaeon *Sulfolobus solfataricus*. Biochemical Journal. 2005;**385**:581-588

[99] Aihara T, Ito T, Yamanaka Y, Noguchi K, Odaka M, Sekine M, et al. Structural and functional characterization of aspartate racemase from the acidothermophilic archaeon *Picrophilus torridus*. Extremophiles. 2016;**20**(4):385-393

[100] Ohara K, Unno H, Oshima Y, Hosoya M, Fujino N, Hirooka K, et al. Structural insights into the low pH adaptation of a unique carboxylesterase from *Ferroplasma*: Altering the pH optima of two carboxylesterases. Journal of Biological Chemistry. 2014;**289**(35):24499-24510

[101] Birrien JL, Zeng X, Jebbar M, Cambon-Bonavita MA, Quérellou J, Oger P, et al. *Pyrococcus yayanosii* sp. nov., an obligate piezophilic hyperthermophilic archaeon isolated from a deep-sea hydrothermal vent. International Journal of Systematic and Evolutionary Microbiology. 2011;**61**(12):2827-2831

[102] Di Giulio M. A comparison of proteins from *Pyrococcus furiosus* and *Pyrococcus abyssi*: Barophily in the physicochemical properties of amino acids and in the genetic code. Gene. 2005;**346**:1-6

[103] Yafremava LS, Di Giulio M, Caetano-Anollés G. Comparative analysis of barophily-related amino acid content in protein domains of *Pyrococcus abyssi* and *Pyrococcus furiosus*. Archaea. 2013;**2013**:680436

[104] Chung YC, Kobayashi T, Kanai H, Akiba T, Kudo T. Purification and properties of extracellular amylase from the hyperthermophilic archaeon *Thermococcus profundus* Dt5432. Applied and Environmental Microbiology. 1995;**61**(4):1502-1506

[105] Pérez-Pomares F, Bautista V, Ferrer J, Pire C, Marhuenda-Egea FC, Bonete MJ. α-Amylase activity from the halophilic archaeon *Haloferax mediterranei*. Extremophiles. 2003;**7**(4):299-306

[106] Kannan Y, Koga Y, Inoue Y, Haruki M, Takagi M, Imanaka T, et al. Active subtilisin-like protease from a hyperthermophilic archaeon in a form with a putative prosequence. Applied and Environmental Microbiology. 2001;**67**(6):2445-2452

[107] Hess M, Katzer M, Antranikian G. Extremely thermostable esterases from the thermoacidophilic euryarchaeon *Picrophilus torridus*. Extremophiles. 2008;**12**(3):351-364

[108] Müller-Santos M, de Souza EM, Pedrosa Fde O, Mitchell DA, Longhi S, Carrière F, et al. First evidence for the salt-dependent folding and activity of an esterase from the halophilic archaea *Haloarcula marismortui*. Biochimica et Biophysica Acta. 2009;**1791**(8):719-729

[109] Gueguen Y, Rolland JL, Lecompte O, Azam P, Le Romancer G, Flament D, et al. Characterization of two DNA polymerases from the hyperthermophilic euryarchaeon *Pyrococcus abyssi*. European Journal of Biochemistry. 2001;**268**(22):5961-5969

[110] Nakayama M, Kohiyama M. An α-like DNA polymerase from *Halobacterium halobium*. European Journal of Biochemistry. 1985;**152**:293-297

[111] Kang HJ, Uegaki K, Fukada H, Ishikawa K. Improvement of the enzymatic activity of the hyperthermophilic cellulase from *Pyrococcus horikoshii*. Extremophiles. 2007;**11**(2):251-256

[112] Zhang T, Datta S, Eichler J, Ivanova N, Axen SD, Kerfeld CA, et al. Identification of a haloalkaliphilic and thermostable cellulase with improved ionic liquid tolerance. Green Chemistry. 2011;**13**(8):2083-2090

[113] Kengen SW, Luesink EJ, Stams AJ, Zehnder AJ. Purification and characterization of an extremely thermostable β-glucosidase from the hyperthermophilic archaeon *Pyrococcus furiosus*. European Journal of Biochemistry. 1993;**213**(1):305-312

[114] Angelov A, Putyrski M, Liebl W. Molecular and biochemical characterization of α-glucosidase and α-mannosidase and their clustered genes from the thermoacidophilic archaeon *Picrophilus torridus*. Journal of Bacteriology. 2006;**188**(20):7123-7131

[115] Synowiecki J, Maciunska J. Isolation and some properties of the thermostable beta-galactosidase of *Pyrococcus woesei* expressed in *Escherichia coli*. Journal of Food Biochemistry. 2002;**26**(1):49-62

[116] Holmes ML, Scopes RK, Moritz RL, Simpson RJ, Englert C, Pfeifer F, et al. Purification and analysis of an extremely halophilic beta-galactosidase from *Haloferax alicantei*. Biochimica et Biophysica Acta. 1997;**1337**(2):276-286

[117] Murphy J. A study of β-galactosidases from thermoacidophiles [doctoral thesis]. University of Limerick; 2013. Available from: http://hdl.handle.net/10344/3609 [Accessed: 2016-12-26]

[118] Karan R, Capes MD, DasSarma P, DasSarma S. Cloning, overexpression, purification, and characterization of a polyextremophilic β-galactosidase from the Antarctic haloarchaeon *Halorubrum lacusprofundi*. BMC Biotechnology. 2013;**13**(1):3

[119] Antoine E, Rolland J-L, Raffin J-P, Dietrich J. Cloning and over-expression in *Escherichia coli* of the gene encoding NADPH group III alcohol dehydrogenase from *Thermococcus hydrothermalis*. European Journal of Biochemistry. 1999;**264**:880-889

[120] Timpson LM, Liliensiek AK, Alsafadi D, Cassidy J, Sharkey MA, Liddell S, et al. A comparison of two novel alcohol dehydrogenase enzymes (ADH1 and ADH2) from the extreme halophile *Haloferax volcanii*. Applied Microbiology and Biotechnology. 2013;**97**(1):195-203

[121] Marino-Marmolejo EN, De León-Rodríguez A, de la Rosa APB, Santos L. Heterologous expression and characterization of an alcohol dehydrogenase from the archeon *Thermoplasma acidophilum*. Molecular Biotechnology. 2009;**42**(1):61-67

[122] Alquéres SMC, Branco RV, Freire DMG, Alves TLM, Martins OB, Almeida RV. Characterization of the recombinant thermostable lipase (Pf2001) from *Pyrococcus furiosus*: Effects of Thioredoxin Fusion Tag and Triton X-100. Enzyme Research. 2011;**2011**:316939

[123] Boutaiba S, Bhatnagar T, Hacene H, Mitchell DA, Baratti JC. Preliminary characterisation of a lipolytic activity from an extremely halophilic archaeon, *Natronococcus* sp. Journal of Molecular Catalysis B: Enzymatic. 2006;**41**(1-2):21-26

[124] Gardner WL, Whitman WB. Expression vectors for *Methanococcus maripaludis*: Overexpression of acetohydroxyacid synthase and β-galactosidase. Genetics. 1999;**152**(4): 1439-1447

[125] O'Connor EM, Shand RF. Halocins and sulfolobicins: The emerging story of archaeal protein and peptide antibiotics. Journal of Industrial Microbiology & Biotechnology. 2002;**28**(1):23-31

[126] Meseguer I, Torreblanca M, Konishi T. Specific inhibition of the halobacterial Na^+/H^+ antiporter by halocin H6. Journal of Biological Chemistry. 1995;**270**:6450-6455

[127] Asker D, Ohta Y. *Haloferax alexandrinus* sp. nov., an extremely halophilic canthaxanthin-producing archaeon from a solar saltern in Alexandria (Egypt). International Journal of Systematic and Evolutionary Microbiology. 2002;**52**(3):729-738

[128] Choquet CG, Patel GB, Sprott GD, Beveridge TJ. Stability of pressure-extrudes liposomes made from archaeobacterial ether lipids. Applied Microbiology and Biotechnology. 1994;**42**(2-3):375-384

Archaebiotics: Archaea as Pharmabiotics for Treating Chronic Disease in Humans?

Wajdi Ben Hania, Nathalie Ballet,
Pascal Vandeckerkove, Bernard Ollivier,
Paul W. O'Toole and Jean-François Brugère

Additional information is available at the end of the chapter

http://dx.doi.org/10.5772/intechopen.69945

Abstract

Recent findings highlight the role of the human gut microbiota in various disorders. For example, atherosclerosis frequently seems to be the consequence of gut microbiota–derived metabolism of some dietary components. Pharmabiotics (i.e., live/dead microbes and microbe-derived substances) and probiotics (live microorganisms with a health benefit when administered in adequate amounts) are a means to counteract these deleterious effects. Among the latter, microbes now being used or, being currently developed, are bacteria and eukaryotes (yeasts), so omitting the third domain of life—the archaea, despite their unique properties that could be of great interest to human health. Here, we promote the idea that some specific archaea are potential next-generation probiotics. This is based on an innovative example of the bioremediation of a gut microbial metabolite. Indeed, besides the fact that they are archaea (i.e. originating from a domain of life from which no pathogens of humans/animals/plants are currently known), they are rationally selected based on (i) being naturally human-hosted, (ii) having a unique metabolism not performed by other human gut microbes, (iii) depleting a deleterious atherogenic compound generated by the human gut microbiota and (iv) generating a health inert gas.

Keywords: archaea, atherosclerosis, cardiovascular disease, methanogens, *Methanomassiliicoccales*, next-generation probiotics, trimethylamine (TMA), trimethylamine oxide (TMAO), trimethylaminuria (TMAU)

1. Introduction

The human intestinal tract is populated with an important number of microbes, which until recently, were believed to account for 10-fold more than the number of human cells [1], but now more likely being equivalent [2]. This contributes to the recent view of humans and other mammals as being metaorganisms. This microbial community is described as the human gut microbiota whose collective genomes form the gut microbiome with about 100-fold the number of human genes [3, 4]. It possesses specific functions leading one consider it as an active organ which influences multiple functions of the human host [5]. Moreover, its composition is different among individuals, resulting and being dependent on various factors: among them, one can cite the delivery mode at birth (i.e. vaginal vs. caesarean [6]), genetics [7] and environmental factors encompassing drug use and diet [8]. The human gut microbiota is typically composed of about 400 different bacterial species (designated as 'operational taxonomic units', (OTUs)) from a repertory of more than 1.000 OTUs [3, 4, 8, 9]. However, if bacteria are the main constituents of the gut microbiota, it is well known that besides viruses, the two other domains of life (i.e. archaea and eukaryota) are also normal constituents of this microbial community. Archaea represent the second most important group of microbes, in number, with a mean of 1.5% of the microbiota as recently determined from metagenomics studies on large cohorts [9] (**Figure 1**).

Among the various roles attributed to the gut microbiota, it acts as a barrier against colonization of pathogens and for the development and maintenance of the gut epithelium and its structural integrity. Also, it modulates the immune system by the continuous interplay with the host immune system. Lastly, it participates in host nutrient metabolism (which is also extended to drugs and xenobiotics) by enriching energy and compound retrieval from nutrients. It encompasses, but is not limited, to the synthesis of vitamins and the hydrolysis and fermentation of organic matter (e.g. indigestible dietary fibre), leading to the production of short-chain fatty acids (SCFA) [10]. The latter accounts for about 5–10% of the overall energy harvested by host from diet [11].

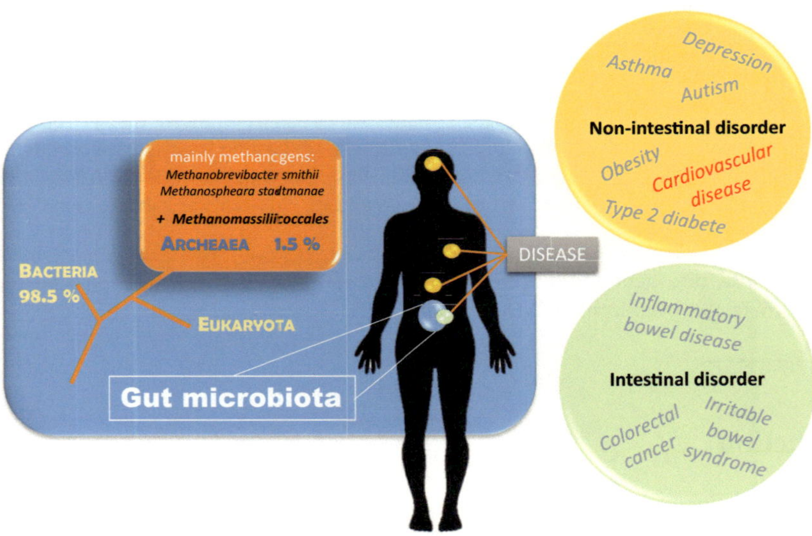

Figure 1. The human gut microbiota, its archaeal component and its role in various disorders, sometimes linked to the gastrointestinal tract (lower right circle), sometimes to other locations (upper right circle).

To date, a close link between the gut microbiota and digestive health has been reported and documented (**Figure 1**). It plays an important role in various digestive disorders [12, 13], like colon carcinogenesis [14], irritable bowel syndrome (IBS) [15] and inflammatory bowel diseases (IBD) encompassing Crohn's disease and ulcerative colitis [16]. On first thought surprising, it is also linked to non-digestive diseases encompassing type 1 and 2 diabetes (T1D and T2D) and obesity, as well as conditions such as asthma, autism and depression [10, 13]. It is also linked to cardiovascular disease (CVD) which will be described in more detail below. Based on these facts, if the microbiota or one of its components is the causing agent of disease, maintaining a healthy microbiota or restoring the microbiota from a dysbiosis state to a normobiosis state should improve health or prevent disorders. Pharmabiotics represent one of the ways by which this can be achieved [17].

In the early twentieth century, Eli Metchnikoff proposed the probiotic concept based on the observation that consuming host-friendly bacteria as done by Bulgarians, i.e. the bacteria found in their yogurts, led to improved health and delayed senility in this population [18]. Probiotics are defined by the World Health Organization (WHO), and the Food and Agricultural Organization (FAO), as 'live microorganisms which, when administered in adequate amounts, confer a health benefit on the host'. Hence, based on this definition, probiotics are microbes that can originate from sources other than food. Based on a rational design inferred from the causation of the disorder, in this chapter, we introduce a new strategic way for discovering new probiotics by highlighting the role that some archaea could play in the human gut. Indeed, one group of archaea found in humans can convert a deleterious compound of gut bacterial dietary metabolism. This bioremediation leads to methane (CH_4), which is considered to be inert for health in the human gut. Therefore, these archaea could become a source of the next generation pharmabiotics, i.e. archaebiotics, originating from the normal composition of the human gut. To date, neither probiotic nor pathogenic microorganisms have been determined to exist in the archaeal domain.

2. Diet, gut microbiota and a particularly deleterious plasma compound

Our health is intimately linked to what we eat. The diet itself may contain deleterious compounds; it may also contain initially neutral or even beneficial nutrients that may become deleterious after being metabolized by our gut microbiota. Cardiovascular disease (CVD) is representative of this two-sided effect. The example below will highlight one of the roles in gut microbiota/diet co-participation. CVD is the leading cause of death according to WHO (2012), corresponding to more than 17 million deaths every year, about one-third of all deaths. A significant part results in the development of atheromatous plaques, an accumulation of lipids and adipose tissue (in particular cholesterol), complex carbohydrates/fibrous connective tissues, minerals and cells (macrophages) on the inner layer of arterial walls. Recognized biological risks are hypertension, chronic hyperglycaemia, hyperlipidaemia and overweight/obesity. Only one fifth of CVD seems to originate from genetic factors, while environment alone, or in combination with genetics likely accounts for all other cases [19]. Among environmental factors which encompass diet, it is very difficult to determine which nutrient(s) specifically act on atherosclerosis development [20]. However, in 2011, one compound was identified in blood that was intimately linked to CVD and whose origin was associated with various ingredients and nutrients from diet [21].

2.1. Trimethylamine oxide and atherosclerosis

In 2011, the Stanley Hazen's laboratory (Cleveland clinic, Cleveland, USA) used a systematic approach and analysed plasma metabolites from a learning cohort of 100 patients with variable CVD risks. They succeeded in determining three different molecules that were significantly present at higher levels in high-risk subjects; trimethylamine *N*-oxide (TMAO), betaine and choline were linked to CVD [21]. Interestingly, these three compounds may have the same alimentary origin that we will discuss below. Results obtained from this learning cohort were successfully used on a large validation cohort of 1876 subjects [21]. Also, an extension to 4000 subjects indicated that plasma TMAO (pTMAO) levels alone were able to predict a 2.5-fold increase of major adverse cardiac events (MACE) at 2 years [22]. Moreover, using this high-value risk factor for prognostics, the authors showed a direct implication of TMAO, or of its precursors, in the creation and development of atheromatous plaque. Studies done *in vitro* and with animal models ($ApoE^{-/-}$ mice) showed a role at the intestinal level (alteration of the cholesterol reverse transport through biliary acids); at the hepatic level (modification of the quantity and composition of the biliary acids pool) and at the arterial level (inflammation, differentiation of macrophages into cholesterol containing foam cells that bind to the atheromatous plaque). All of this contributes to atherosclerosis. Moreover, pTMAO enhances platelet hyperactivity therefore increasing the thrombosis risk [23], at least in mice.

2.2. Trimethylamine oxide and other disorders

Besides atherosclerosis, trimethylamine oxide (TMAO) has been linked to several other important disorders, which does not necessarily mean that TMAO may cause the development of the disease. Among them, chronic kidney disease (CKD) and, more specifically, the severity of renal dysfunction are strongly associated with the level of pTMAO [24]. This is likely attributable to deficiencies in glomerular filtration which leads to altered increase clearance of pTMAO (see Section 2.3.) and accumulation of TMAO in blood [25]. However, there are several lines of evidence that pTMAO itself also contributes directly to progressive renal fibrosis, at least in animals [26].

Also, type 2 diabetes (T2D) is associated with higher pTMAO levels [27], but until now, it is still unclear if this is due to a confounding action with glycaemic control or renal function. Interestingly however, various mice T2D models showed that one key liver enzyme implicated in the generation of TMA (FMO3, see Section 2.3.) was regulated by insulin [28].

Other disorders analysed so far also encompass colorectal cancer (CRC), for which data remain unclear; a study reported the building of epigenetic interaction networks from data of interactions between chemicals and genes, between diseases and genes and between proteins [29]. This approach was validated by an efficient detection of the known link between TMAO and CVD; it also revealed a stronger genetic link between TMAO and CRC as well as one weaker with metabolic syndromes. The link between TMAO and the risk of CRC was also established in post-menopausal women [30]. However, all of these results need confirmations/validations, and more importantly, if pTMAO is linked, it is a causing agent.

2.3. Origin of plasma trimethylamine oxide

In order to prevent these disorders, it is essential to determine the plasma origin of the above mentioned and linked molecules: betaine, choline, and more specifically, trimethylamine oxide (TMAO). People given a specific meal (eggs, see below) showed a rise of TMAO in their plasma (pTMAO). Interestingly, after broad-spectrum antibiotic treatment, leading to the eradication of as much as possible gut microbes, pTMAO disappeared after the same meal and reappeared a few weeks after the cessation of the antibiotics treatment, i.e. when the gut microbiota had recovered [22]. Therefore, pTMAO levels are dependent on the nature of the nutrients and of the gut microbiota. Nutrients are provided by a broad alimentary range of sources; and, among them, TMAO itself which is used as an osmoregulant in many marine life forms and is consequently found in some seafood. Much more studied are choline and phosphatidylcholine (PC, also referred as lecithin), which are found in eggs, red meat, fishes, cheese, and some vegetables [31, 32]. It also encompasses L-carnitine which is found mainly in red meat and recently in some energizing drinks. When ingested, a fraction of dietary choline/PC and L-carnitine reaches gut microbes which can metabolize them into trimethylamine (TMA). The metabolic activity of anaerobic organisms is still poorly understood and the bacterial enzymes which can convert these compounds into TMA have only recently been determined [33–36]. TMAO is also metabolized into TMA in the gut by bacteria. **Figure 2** indicates the different pathways that lead to TMA in the gut.

Importantly, the genes encoding these various enzymes are for the most part not specific to a bacterial lineage, and horizontal gene transfers have occurred during evolution. As a consequence, based on strictly microbial composition, i.e. 16S amplicon sequencing, this currently impairs ways to determine the levels of capability of gut microbiota to deal with these compounds in generating TMA. However, two recent papers showed that it is possible to decipher this capability from metagenomics sequencing data (sequencing of whole microbial DNA from gut/faecal microbiota) by seeking and counting reads corresponding to marker genes in these pathways [37, 38].

The discussed metabolic pathways result in TMA in the gut due to the activity of the microbiota. This forms the unique way for the accumulation of TMA in the digestive tract as TMA is not ingested by itself through the diet. In fact, this molecule has a very repulsive odour for humans as it corresponds to the odour of rotten fish, for which humans are particularly sensitive (see Section 2.4.). TMA is absorbed by the gut epithelium, diffuses and reaches the portal vein. It is next oxidized in the liver by monooxygenases, more specifically the hepatic flavin–containing monooxygenase 3 (FMO3), resulting in pTMAO. Interestingly, this enzyme is not only transcriptionally regulated by several elements encompassing sex hormones and biliary acids [39, 40] but also by insulin. pTMAO is excreted via the kidneys into urine. Indeed, TMAO has higher renal clearance than urea and creatinine in healthy humans [25]. However, as previously mentioned, impaired renal function leads to higher pTMAO levels as observed in subjects suffering from chronic kidney disease (CKD) [24].

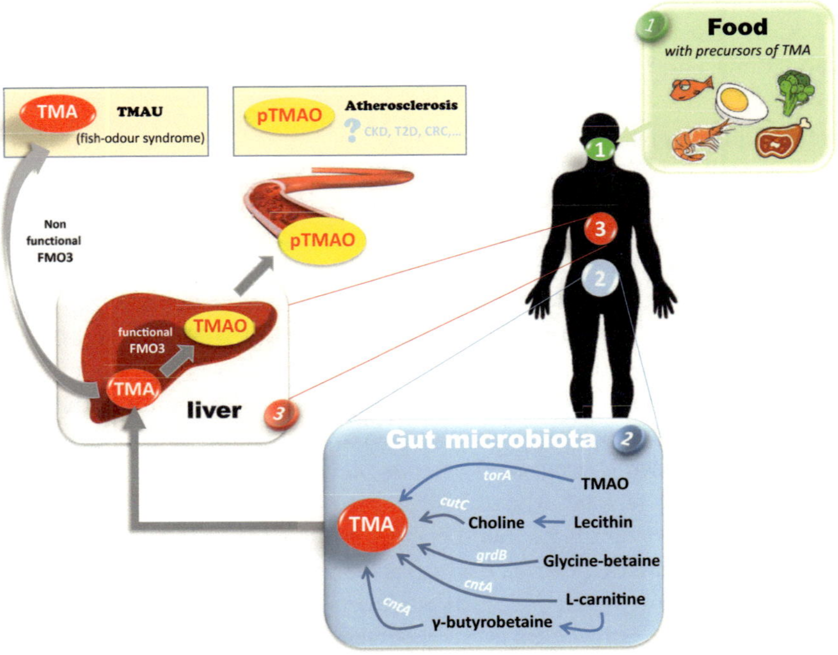

Figure 2. Origin, fate and implication of trimethylamine TMA and trimethylamine oxide TMAO in various disorders through the synthesis of TMA by the human gut microbiota. (1) various kinds of food contain nutrients like TMAO, lecithin, choline and L-carnitine. These nutrients come into contact with various gut microbes (2) that are differentially present among individuals. Some of these gut bacteria can metabolize these nutrients into TMA with dedicated enzymes whose encoding genes are indicated in italics. The TMA generated is absorbed from the gut into the portal vein from which it reaches the liver (3). Some people lack an efficient TMA oxidizing activity through the flavin-containing monooxygenase 3 (upper part, left box), either because of a genetic defect or an acquired one, through hepatic dysfunctions/down-regulation of FMO3 expression: this leads to TMA in blood, which can diffuse in any body fluid from which it is eliminated. This leads to trimethylaminuria (TMAU) or fish-odour syndrome. In a more general case, FMO3 activity is sufficient enough to oxidize TMA into TMAO, which enters the circulation (pTMAO). This compound is deleterious and leads through various mechanisms to atherosclerosis and possibly also chronic kidney disease (CKD), type 2 diabetes (T2D) and colorectal cancer (CRC) (upper central box).

2.4. The peculiar case of trimethylaminuria

Trimethylaminuria (TMAU) is a metabolic disorder leading to a TMA/TMAO ratio in urine above 5%, indicating a deficiency in liver oxidative processing of TMA [41, 42]. This is likely an under-recognized and underdiagnosed disease. It has important psychological and social concerns for people suffering from this metabolic disorder. While TMA is partly excreted in the urine, it is also eliminated in the breath and sweat; affected people have a rotten-fish odour which is very unpleasant. Humans are very sensitive to the odour, probably a remnant of our evolution which prevents us from eating spoiled fish. This fish-odour syndrome (the other name for TMAU) is caused by a deficiency in functional FMO3. This is mainly a genetic disorder (autosomal recessive) corresponding to a rare inborn disease, with about 0.5–1.0% of the UK population being heterozygous carriers in the white UK population [43–45]. Therefore, it can be presumed that about 1 on 40,000 subjects is affected in Great Britain. Also, temporary symptoms have been described, resulting in secondary/acquired TMAU: this is due to the regulation of the FMO3 (sex hormone dependant), transient liver deficiencies (e.g. viral hepatitis), or overload of dietary precursors of TMA by gut microbes [44, 46]

2.5. Strategy to lower plasma trimethylamine oxide

In consequence, lowering plasma trimethylamine oxide (pTMAO) levels is a goal in reaching the prevention of, at least partially, the disorders discussed above and more specifically atherosclerosis. Theoretically, three main targets may be considered: first, this can be achieved by reducing the precursors of pTMAO that are found in diet. Second, alteration of the gut microbiota composition can modify its metabolic behaviour thereby decreasing the synthesis of intestinal TMA from dietary precursors. Third, intestinal TMA that has been synthesized can be diverted from its hepatic oxidation into TMAO. If we have a more detailed look at each of these possibilities, most of them are unrealistic and/or hazardous for humans.

2.5.1. Decreasing TMAO precursors from diet

There are many concerns about trying to limit the contribution of TMAO precursors in diet. First, it seems unrealistic for several reasons. As noted previously, there are not one but several potential precursors which include lecithin, choline, L-carnitine, and TMAO. Moreover, these nutrients are found in a broad diversity of foods, which makes the formulation of ingredients and meals difficult; this has also to be considered within cultural/individual backgrounds. Also, in this peculiar case where the link between nutrients and pTMAO relies on the gut microbiota composition, which is individual specific, it is very difficult to promote some foods rather than others knowing that not all individuals would be affected in the same way.

However, the concerns over dietary TMAO precursor removal are frustrating considering the main drawback of such a proposition. First, many foods are recognized as health promoting despite the fact that they contain TMAO precursors. For example, fish consumption is recommended twice a week for people at risk for coronary heart disease due the presence of omega-3 fatty acids like eicosapentaenoic acid (EPA) and docosahexaenoic acid (DHA) (American Heart Association recommendations) [47]. TMAO and choline/lecithin can be consumed in large amounts via these diets. Second, and much more important, the precursors of pTMAO are highly desirable in sufficient amounts for many other roles they play in our body, and their limitations could lead inversely to other disorders. As a prime example, such recommendations could lead to choline deficiencies, whose daily intake has been established to be between 425 and 550 mg/day, respectively, for women and men in the United States. These levels are required to avoid the induction of major cognitive complications and liver disease such as hepatic steatosis [48–50].

2.5.2. Decreasing intestinal TMA synthesis

Decreasing TMA synthesis in the gut by the microbiota would result in less TMA reaching the liver where it is converted into deleterious pTMAO. This goal may be achieved by several ways, for example, the use of medication, prebiotics, probiotics and faecal microbiota transplantation (FMT). To our knowledge, there is no evidence, to date, of a probiotic with activity that is capable of reducing TMA synthesis in the gut; but, the use of probiotics would be a fine strategy due to its potential for large-scale use. FMT is also very promising as it is used for several disorders that are associated by a dysbiosis of the gut microbiota and could be of the highest interest in this case. However, this technique is still in its infancy and long-term consequence/maintenance of a supposed 'good' microbiota is unknown. In fact, it seems that such maintenance is rather an 'ecological agreement' between the recipient (its physiology/genetics/diet/gut microbiota) and the faecal microbial transplant, leading to a mixed microbiota of host/donor. It cannot be assumed that microbes leading to TMA will be eradicated or at least drastically lowered. Therefore, such an intervention may have to be conducted frequently and at a large scale. This approach relies on limited donors, and there is an absence of a biotechnological way to amplify such complex microbiota. Also, there is still a lack of an efficient safety procedure concerning the donor at the moment of transplantation due to the absence of an efficient way to preserve the faecal microbiota; increasing donors and repeating the process could lead to an increase of the risk of transmission of infectious diseases by viruses or pathogenic bacteria.

Prebiotics is another way to support beneficial microbes of the gut. It can be noted that compliance to a Mediterranean diet (which is known to decrease CVD risks) leads to lower pTMAO levels [51], lending support to the fact that some elements of this kind of diet may contain beneficial factors for this purpose. Interestingly, it has been shown recently that resveratrol, a natural phytoalexin found notably in grapes and i.e. the Mediterranean diet has a prebiotic effect; it remodels the gut microbiota in a beneficial way (encompassing an increase of bile acids by *de novo* synthesis in the liver) and leads to a decrease of pTMAO [52].

Finally, medication is another way by which the gut microbiota may be remodelled. At the extreme, the use of antibiotics provides an efficient way to this goal, it is sometimes used to treat TMAU patients [42]. This approach proves that TMA synthesis can be efficiently but temporarily curtailed; it seems, however, unreasonable to propose the large-scale use of broad spectrum antibiotics for this purpose, or its repeated use in affected individuals. Ideally, the use of a drug or a combination of drugs would have a more specific action, either by targeting bacteria from groups that are known to potentially produce TMA or better by targeting the bacterial enzymes involved in TMA synthesis. A very promising drug has been recently described, 3,3-dimethyl-1-butanol (DMB) [53]. This compound is a substrate analogue of choline that inhibits TMA-lyases, the bacterial enzyme family that converts several substrates into TMA. It is not only active against the synthesis of TMA from choline, but also from L-carnitine, at least in some bacterial groups and does not seem to have any lethal effect on these bacteria. Therefore, its use should not lead to dramatic changes in the microbiota constitution. Also, interestingly, DMB is naturally found in components of the Mediterranean diet (olive oils, red wines) [54]. It remains however to be determined to which extent DMB use will decrease pTMAO. In addition, another drug was described a few years ago, already known to have clinically cardioprotective effects, supposedly by lowering L-carnitine content in the body [55]. This compound, meldonium (also referred as mildronate, formally 3-(2,2,2-trimethylhydrazinium) propionate dehydrate), has been shown to lower pTMAO [56] which may be due partly on the prevention of bacterial L-carnitine use [57].

2.5.3. Preventing TMA oxidation into TMAO by the liver

Once TMA has been generated by the microbiota in the gut, one can conceivably try to lower its oxidation into pTMAO by host FMO3 enzymes in the liver. Among various solutions, one could focus on the inhibition of FMO3. However, this would (i) likely lead to deleterious effects by affecting the oxidation/detoxification of other compounds and (ii) allow TMA to enter the general circulation at high amounts; symptoms similar to TMAU would appear, i.e. a rotten fish odour emanating from the subjects. Therefore, alternatives need to be found that lower TMA availability in the gut. While it seems unrealistic to inhibit specifically its absorption by acting on epithelial transporters, charcoal is sometimes efficiently used by TMAU patients [42], which leads to a decrease of symptoms by increasing TMA excretion in faeces. Therefore, this likely lowers TMA in body fluids in these patients, and it can reasonably be assumed that TMA reaching the liver would be lowered in non-TMAU patients, and that, in consequence, pTMAO would be lowered. However, it is unclear if this can be applied as a long-term strategy without lowering the absorption of other important intestinal compounds and that could lead to deficiencies.

In summary, it would be of great interest to have a specific agent acting only on intestinal TMA. This could be achieved by a biological system able to convert TMA into inert molecules in a complex environment (the gut and its microbiota) and without danger to humans. While no bacterial species seems suitable, one recently identified group of archaea seems to provide all these properties.

3. Human naturally hosted archaea that prevent plasma trimethylamine oxide formation

Archaea belong to one of the three domains of life [58]. They are unicellular microorganisms distinct from bacteria and eukaryotic cells in regard to evolution and some of their cellular/molecular processes. For example, their cell membrane has a different composition compared to bacteria and eukaryotes [59]. In fact, archaea can be characterized as cells looking like bacteria but having cellular, molecular and genetics characteristics of eukaryotes but with some differences. One archaeal group recently identified (*Lokiarchaeota*) has been proposed to be at the origin of eukaryote evolutionary divergence, and so, perhaps, a direct ancestor of our own cells [60]. Also, the domain *Archaea* contains microbes with a unique mechanism by which they derive energy not found anywhere else in other life forms, i.e. methanogenesis [61]. Some methanogenic archaea are found as natural components of the gut microbiota [62], where they are principal methane producers. So far also, no pathogens are known among the archaea, neither in humans nor in any other animal or plants.

3.1. A recently discovered archaeal lineage primarily recovered from human stools that thrived in various environments

About a decade ago, we revealed the existence of unknown archaea in the faecal microbiota of some humans [63, 64], with clues that they were methanogens even if belonging to a lineage

(*Thermoplasmata*) with no other known methanogens. Up to now, only one member has been isolated in pure culture. *Methanomassiliicoccus (Mmc.) luminyensis* strain B10 was isolated by the joint efforts of two laboratories [65], which lead to the creation of a new methanogenic archaeal order named *Methanomassiliicoccales* [66]. Also, we have currently a highly enriched culture with another strain from this order which shows only 89% nucleotide identity for its 16S rRNA compared to *Mmc. luminyensis* B10. It has been named *Ca.* Methanomethylophilus alvus Mx1201. These two strains were obtained from human faecal samples. Phylogenetic data based on a DNA survey revealed that this group of methanogens is found in various ecosystems [67, 68]. These anaerobic environments encompass notably seafloor, wetlands, biogas fermenters, etc. but also the gastrointestinal tract of a broad variety of animals. Among them, one can cite insects like termites [69], ruminants [68, 70–73], and humans [62–65, 74]. Very interestingly, three clusters of *Methanomassiliicoccales* have been identified [67, 68], reflecting the environmental source of sampling. One large cluster of neighbouring 16S and/or *mcrA* (a molecular marker of methanogens) sequences corresponds to members almost exclusively retrieved from gastrointestinal tracts. *Ca.* Methanomethylophilus alvus Mx1201 belongs to this cluster, also referred as the host-associated- or Gastro-Intestinal Tract (GIT) clade. A second cluster contains members retrieved from GIT as well as anaerobic environments like soils or freshwater lakes, etc. and is therefore named the mixed cluster, to which *Methanomassiliicoccus* spp. belongs. Finally, the third clade is formed of members exclusively recovered from nondigestive environments, at least until now [67, 68].

Still little is known about these archaea, except for the fact that they are methanogens with a peculiar metabolism [72, 75, 76]. Their biology is mainly known from genomic studies with recent new data (**Table 1**). Also, microbiological studies have been possible on enrichment

Name	Clade	Host/ Environment	Isolate$	TMA use*	References
***Mmc. luminyensis* B10**	Mixed	Human	Y	Y (G-AE)	Gorlas et al. [93]; Borrel et al. [67, 84]; Brugère et al. [80]
***Ca.* Mmp. alvus Mx1201**	Digestive	Human	-	Y (G-EE)	Borrel et al. [75]
***Ca.* Mmc. intestinalis Issoire Mx1**	Mixed	Human	-	Y (G)	Borrel et al. [67, 84]
***Ca.* Methanoplasma termitum**	Digestive	Termite	-	N (G-EE)	Lang et al. [77]
RumEn MG1–RumEn MG2	Digestive	Bovine	-	Y (G)	Sollinger et al. [68]
ISO4-G1	Digestive	Sheep	-	Y (G)	Kelly et al. [94]
ISO4-H5	Digestive	Sheep	-	Y (G)	Li et al. [95]
***Ca.* Mmp. sp. 1R26**	Digestive	Bovine	-	Y (G)	Noel et al. [96]

Notes: $Y refers to a *Methanomassiliicoccales* strain that has been obtained in pure culture.

*Y and N signify, respectively, that the strain can use (Y) or not use (N) TMA as a methanogenesis substrate, based on genomic evidence (G), experimental evidence with enriched culture (EE) or axenic culture (AE).

Table 1. Available genomic data from *Methanomassiliicoccales* (end of year 2016).

cultures with the isolate *Mmc. luminyensis* B10 [65]. However, the highly enriched culture of *Ca.* Methanomethylophilus alvus Mx1201 from the host-associated clade has already helped to characterize one potential health-related metabolic property.

3.2. TMA remediation into methane by some *Methanomassiliicoccales*

3.2.1. *Original methanogens with unique biological property*

The biological features, mainly deciphered from genomic data, have revealed several uncommon points. Among them, it is likely that they possess two cellular membranes [77], whose composition is typical of other archaea; their phospholipids are indeed composed of L-glycerol (instead of D-glycerol as observed in bacterial and eukaryotic phospholipids) and of isoprenoid side-branch chains (instead of fatty acids as in the two other domains of life). They are linked to L-glycerol by an ether bond, instead of an ester bond. However, the cell membranes of *Mmc. luminyensis* are somewhat different from known archaeal membranes. There are chemically important nuances; some tetraether lipids (typically two L-glycerols linked by isoprenoid chains at both sides and thus not forming a two-layer membrane) are composed of one butanetriol or one pentanetriol replacing one L-glycerol [78]. Also, the processes that drive energy acquisition from methanogenesis (electron-transport and proton extraction outside the cell to be used as a proton motive force linked to ATP synthesis) are different from other methanogens [76, 77, 79] and are not currently fully understood.

However, the other important feature is their ability to synthesize and incorporate a specific unusual amino-acid, pyrrolysine (IUAB nomenclature: Pyl, O) during the translation of mRNAs [76, 80]. This incorporation is mediated by a dedicated tRNA, whose particularity, besides its size, is to recognize the *amber* codon UAG, which is usually one of the three nonsense codons (**Figure 3**). This '22nd amino-acid' is restricted to specific organisms (methanogens of the taxonomic family *Methanosarcinaceae* and about 20 different bacterial species) and to specific proteins, the methyl transferases that can capture methyl groups in methylamines (i.e. monomethylamine (MMA), dimethylamine (DMA) and trimethylamine (TMA)). The reader can find more information about this amino acid and the mechanisms underlying its incorporation into proteins, at least in bacteria, in various excellent articles and reviews [81–83].

3.2.2. *Genomic data indicating a TMA remediation in some but not all members of Methanomassiliicoccales*

Analysis of the genome of *Ca.* Methanomethylophilus alvus strain Mx1201 [75] and *Ca.* Methanomassiliicoccus intestinalis strain Issoire Mx01 [84] revealed that these *Methanomassiliicoccales* could use methylamines as substrates for their methanogenesis. Comparative genomic analysis with the genome of *Mmc. luminyensis* revealed that it should also be the case for this unique isolate available at this time [76]. Indeed, all the genes necessary for this metabolism were present, sometimes at more than one copy each. Here, we will focus on the genome of *Ca.* Methanomethylophilus alvus strain Mx1201 as it specifically illustrates this point. As shown in **Figure 3**, the genes encoding methyltransferases and associated proteins, together with the genes necessary for methane release (methyl-coM reductase (MCR)) are present; this encompasses genes for the use of MMA

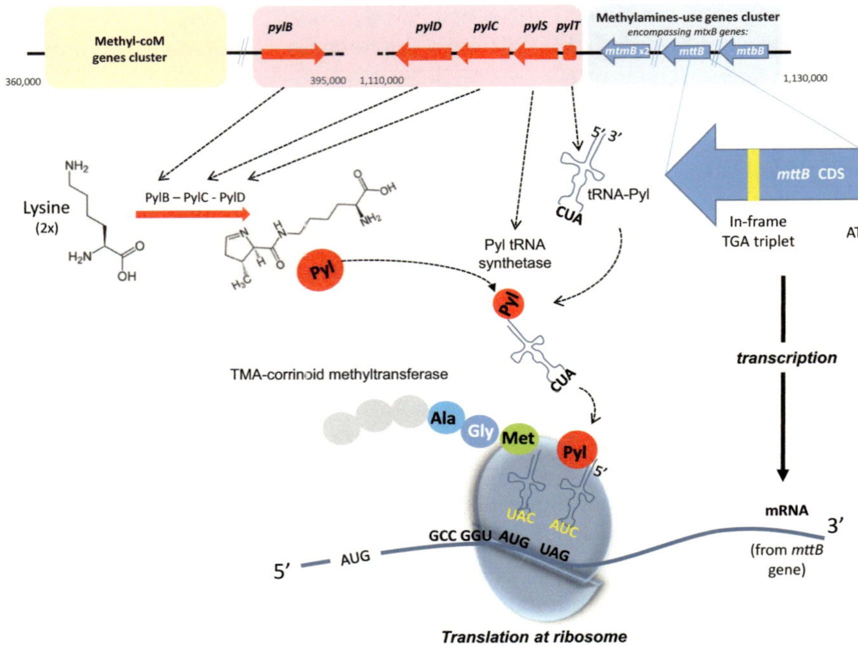

Figure 3. Synthesis mechanism of functional, pyrrolysine-containing TMA-corrinoid methyltransferase. The genetic loci of important genes involved in H_2-dependant methanogenesis using TMA as a substrate are given in the upper part of the figure, taking *Ca.* Methanomethylophilus alvus Mx1201 as an example. Genes involved in the synthesis and translational use of Pyl are indicated by arrows in the upper central box. It encompasses *pylB* which is genetically linked to the genes encoding the methyl-coM reductase (MCR, upper left box), an essential enzyme of methanogenesis necessary for the ultimate reaction in any methanogenic pathway. It also encompasses four other genes that neighbour genes implicated in the use of methylamines (MMA, DMA and TMA; upper right box). Among them, only genes encoding methylamines-corrinoid methyltransferases are shown (*mtxB*), with a focus (right part) made on the *mttB* CDS (coding DNA sequence) which encodes TMA-corrinoid methyltransferase. A TGA triplet is found in its reading frame. Pyrrolysine originates from two lysines using three enzymes encoded by *pylB, C* and *D*. A specific Pyl-tRNA bearing a CUA anticodon is synthesized by transcription of *pylT*. It is further charged with pyrrolysine by specific enzymatic activity of a dedicated AA-tRNA synthetase encoded by the *pylS* gene. After transcription of the *mttB* gene, the corresponding mRNA is translated on ribosomes (lower part of the figure). The *amber* codon UAG, instead of being interpreted as a translational stop, is instead recognized by Pyl-tRNA, which leads to the continuation of translation and the incorporation of Pyl into the TMA-corrinoid methyltransferase, which is necessary for its biological activity.

(*mtm* genes), DMA (*mtb* genes) and TMA (*mtt* genes). Also, the genes for the use of methanol for methanogenesis (*mta* genes) are present. At the current stage of our investigations, data seem to indicate that this species is limited to four possible substrates, namely methanol, MMA, DMA and TMA, at least one of them being essential for its life. In fact, all other potential pathways for methanogenesis are absent, as genomes sequenced to date show a complete lack of genes involved in methanogenesis from $CO_2 + H_2$ (hydrogenotrophic methanogenesis) and from acetate (aceticlastic methanogenesis pathways) [68, 76, 77]. Considering methylamines, their use is dependant of the ability of the organism to encode Pyl: as previously mentioned, this is the case, at least for *Ca.* Methanomethylophilus alvus, *Mmc. luminyensis* and *Ca.* Mmc. intestinalis. However, the example of *Ca.* Methanomethylophilus alvus is very interesting; instead being grouped in one operon as typically found in other Pyl-coding organisms, the *pyl* genes necessary for synthesis and translational incorporation of Pyl (encompassing the gene encoding the *amber* suppressive tRNA) are scattered among two different loci. The gene *pylB* which encodes one enzyme necessary for the biosynthesis of Pyl is found in the vicinity of the genes encoding the essential enzyme of methanogenesis, MCR, while all other *pyl* genes are found in the same locus for genes encoding methyltransferases for the use of MMA, DMA and TMA. This can be interpreted as an evolution which has favoured the linkage of methanogenesis (*mcr* operon), Pyl encoding property and the use of methylamines. This highlights the possible importance of this organism, which lives in the human gut, having the ability to use methylamines.

However, the genetic properties for the use of TMA for methanogenesis are not shared by all *Methanomassiliicoccales* in humans [38]. Currently, available sequence data of *Methanomassiliicoccales* genomes (end of year 2016) also reveal that one termite-hosted *Methanomassiliicoccales* does not carry the *mtt* genes for TMA use [77] (**Table 1**): using enrichment cultures, it showed no growth on TMA or DMA (in presence of H_2, see below) but was able to grow on methanol and MMA (+H_2), as predicted from genomic data [77]. So, one question remains: are there some *Methanomassiliicoccales*, preferably isolated from human GITs for which TMA depletion into methane is demonstrated?

3.2.3. *Experimental evidence that TMA is depleted by some human gut members in presence of H_2*

In addition to experiments that have been conducted with enriched, nonpure cultures, we have been able to show that the isolate from the mixed cluster *Mmp. luminyensis* was able to use methanol as well as MMA and TMA, in presence of H_2, to generate methane [80]. Recently, experiments were also conducted with *Ca.* Methanomethylophilus alvus in enrichment cultures [38]. The results clearly indicated that this strain, obtained from a human faecal sample, is able to use TMA in the presence of H_2. Importantly, H_2 is a gas which is generated in large amounts in the gut by the fermentative metabolism of gut microbes. In order to keep fermentations of high yield, without catabolic repression, it needs to be efficiently removed by hydrogenotrophs, i.e. mainly hydrogenotrophic methanogens, sulphate reducers and bacteria performing reductive acetogenesis. Also, analyses of faecal TMA levels have very recently revealed significant differences of the presence or the absence of *Methanomassiliicoccales* [38]: In fact, in the Irish ELDERMET cohort consisted of older subjects (>64 years of age) [85, 86], subjects had significantly lower TMA concentrations in their stools when harbouring *Methanomassiliicoccales* possessing the genetic behaviour to deplete TMA compared with subjects not carrying *Methanomassiliicoccales*. The significance of this observation was increased when the level of potentially TMA using *Methanomassiliicoccales* was above 10^8 cells/gram of stool than below [38].

4. Conclusion: archaebiotics, next-generation probiotics?

Through these preliminary data, it is very tempting to propose the use of strains like *Ca.* Methanomethylophilus alvus Mx1201 as next-generation probiotics (**Figure 4**). That is, a periodic ingestion of an archaeal strain in a form and dosage that remains to be determined

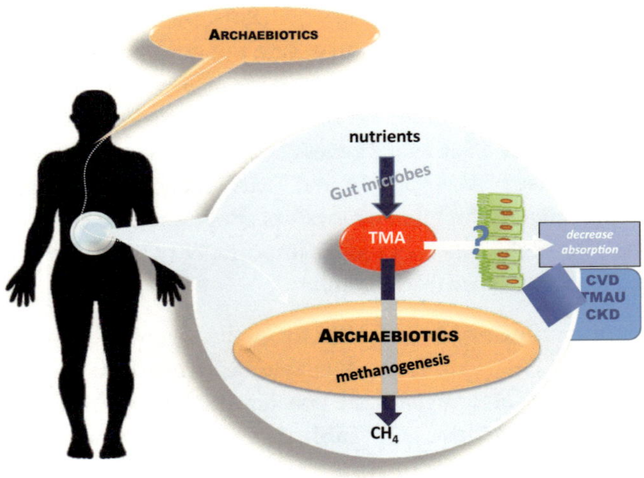

Figure 4. Principle and indications for the use of *Methanomassiliicoccales* as an archaebiotic for depletion of atherogenic trimethylamine TMA. Using the unique property of TMA use by some *Methanomassiliicoccales* and knowing the mechanisms by which pTMAO originates, it is proposed using the human-hosted strain *Ca.* Methanomethylophilus alvus Mx1201 and other rationally selected strains to lower TMA generated by gut microbes directly in the gut/before its absorption. This bioremediation would lead to methane which is considered as a heath-inert intestinal gas. This would, either limit circulating TMA, therefore lowering symptoms of trimethylaminuria, or limit pTMAO levels, therefore preventing, at a minimum, atherosclerosis and chronic kidney disease.

with the aim of preventing at least CVD by limiting the yield of pTMAO. The mechanism relies on the remediation of gut TMA synthesized by gut microbes into a gas (methane) considered as inert to human physiology. Interestingly, this action should also be effective in lowering the symptoms of TMAU. To our knowledge, this is, therefore, a very innovative probiotic design considering that

- Archaea, for which no pathogens are known, had not been considered for probiotics use until now.
- The microorganisms that fit this use are directly selected from human gut microbial inhabitants. They are more prevalent in older people when considering Western countries [38, 64, 74, 87], but they are also highly prevalent in any age group in one Amazonian tribe, the Yanomami hunter-gatherers in Venezuela [88].
- Their selection is based on the knowledge of the mechanisms underlying the pathology and is therefore rationally selected first using simple *in vitro* tests (here, capability of TMA usage).

Importantly, despite lacking definitive proof, it has to be noted that the use of TMA by some human-hosted *Methanomassiliicoccales* is very likely the metabolism they naturally perform in the gut environment. The distribution pattern of the *pyl* genes in the genome of *Ca.* Methanomethylophilus alvus Mx1201 supports this hypothesis (see above). In fact, it is also suspected that this metabolism is the reason for their presence in such an environment; i.e. they occupy an ecological niche that other gut members cannot occupy, and they are highly adapted to this environment. Considering

http://dx.doi.org/10.5772/intechopen.69945

its importance to resisting this host-derived antimicrobial component, the presence of a bile salt hydrolysis gene in *Ca*. Methanomethylophilus alvus Mx1201 from a bacterial lateral gene transfer (LGT) also supports this hypothesis. It should also be considered that this activity has a possible role in CVD prevention by lowering circulating cholesterol [89].

In any case, many more experiments are needed to address the question that some *Methanomas siliicoccales* may be efficiently and safely used in humans. *In vitro* experiments in systems mimicking the gut microbial environment [90, 91] which has been shown to efficiently support methanogens [92] should help to determine the metabolic behaviour of these archaea as well their interactions with other gut microbes. The isolation of a digestive clade member (for example, *Ca*. Methanomethylophilus alvus Mx1201) is therefore an essential and necessary step, before animal and clinical tests.

Acknowledgements

PWOT's laboratory is supported by Science Foundation Ireland through a Centre award to the APC Microbiome Institute (SFI/12/RC/2273). The authors thank Gunnard K. Jacobson from Lesaffre Yeast Corporation/Lesaffre Human Care/USA for English language edition.

Author details

Wajdi Ben Hania[1], Nathalie Ballet[2], Pascal Vandeckerkove[2], Bernard Ollivier[3], Paul W. O'Toole[4] and Jean-François Brugère[1]*

*Address all correspondence to: jf.brugere@udamail.fr

1 Université Clermont-Auvergne, EA-CIDAM, Clermont-Ferrand, France

2 Lesaffre International, Lesaffre Group, Marcq-en-Barœul, France

3 Aix Marseille Université, CNRS, Université de Toulon, IRD, Mediterranean Institute of Oceanography (MIO), Marseille, France

4 School of Microbiology & APC Microbiome Institute, University College Cork, Cork, Ireland

References

[1] Savage DC. Microbial ecology of the gastrointestinal tract. Annual Review of Microbiology. 1977;**31**:107-133

[2] Sender R, Fuchs S, Milo R. Revised estimates for the number of human and bacteria cells in the body. PLoS Biology. 2016;**14**(8):e1002533

[3] Arumugam M, et al. Enterotypes of the human gut microbiome. Nature. 2011;**473**(7346): 174-180

[4] Human Microbiome Project. Structure, function and diversity of the healthy human microbiome. Nature. 2012;**486**(7402):207-214

[5] O'Hara AM, Shanahan F. The gut flora as a forgotten organ. EMBO Reports. 2006;**7**(7): 688-693

[6] Dominguez-Bello MG, et al. Delivery mode shapes the acquisition and structure of the initial microbiota across multiple body habitats in newborns. Proceedings of the National Academy of Sciences of the United States of America. 2010;**107**(26):11971-11975

[7] Goodrich JK, et al. Human genetics shape the gut microbiome. Cell. 2014;**159**(4):789-799

[8] Zhernakova A, et al. Population-based metagenomics analysis reveals markers for gut microbiome composition and diversity. Science. 2016;**352**(6285):565-569

[9] Falony G, et al. Population-level analysis of gut microbiome variation. Science. 2016;**352** (6285):560-564

[10] Clemente JC, et al. The impact of the gut microbiota on human health: An integrative view. Cell. 2012;**148**(6):1258-1270

[11] Bergman EN. Energy contributions of volatile fatty acids from the gastrointestinal tract in various species. Physiological Reviews. 1990;**70**(2):567-590

[12] Guarner F, Malagelada JR. Gut flora in health and disease. Lancet. 2003;**361**(9356):512-519

[13] Marchesi JR, et al. The gut microbiota and host health: A new clinical frontier. Gut. 2016;**65**(2):330-339

[14] Louis P, Hold GL, Flint HJ. The gut microbiota, bacterial metabolites and colorectal cancer. Nature Reviews Microbiology. 2014;**12**(10):661-672

[15] Collins SM. A role for the gut microbiota in IBS. Nature Reviews Gastroenterology & Hepatology. 2014;**11**(8):497-505

[16] Kostic AD, Xavier RJ, Gevers D. The microbiome in inflammatory bowel disease: Current status and the future ahead. Gastroenterology. 2014;**146**(6):1489-1499

[17] Shanahan F, et al. Pharmabiotics: Bioactives from mining host-microbe-dietary interactions. The Functional Foods Revolution. 2009;**1**:1-6

[18] Howell TH. Metchnikoff and prolongation of life. Age and Ageing. 1988;**17**(6):420-421

[19] Ripatti S, et al. A multilocus genetic risk score for coronary heart disease: Case-control and prospective cohort analyses. Lancet. 2010;**376**(9750):1393-400

[20] Freedman LS, et al. Dealing with dietary measurement error in nutritional cohort studies. Journal of the National Cancer Institute. 2011;**103**(14):1086-1092

[21] Wang Z, et al. Gut flora metabolism of phosphatidylcholine promotes cardiovascular disease. Nature. 2011;**472**(7341):57-63

[22] Tang WH, et al. Intestinal microbial metabolism of phosphatidylcholine and cardiovascular risk. The New England Journal of Medicine. 2013;**368**(17):1575-1584

[23] Zhu W, et al. Gut microbial metabolite TMAO enhances platelet hyperreactivity and thrombosis risk. Cell. 2016;**165**(1):111-124

[24] Missailidis C, et al. Serum trimethylamine-N-oxide is strongly related to renal function and predicts outcome in chronic kidney disease. PLoS One. 2016;**11**(1):e0141738

[25] Hai X, et al. Mechanism of prominent trimethylamine oxide (TMAO) accumulation in hemodialysis patients. PLoS One. 2015;**10**(12):e0143731

[26] Tang WW, et al. Gut microbiota-dependent trimethylamine N-oxide (TMAO) pathway contributes to both development of renal insufficiency and mortality risk in chronic kidney disease novelty and significance. Circulation Research. 2015;**116**(3):448-455

[27] Lever M, et al. Betaine and trimethylamine-N-oxide as predictors of cardiovascular outcomes show different patterns in diabetes mellitus: An observational study. PLoS One. 2014;**9**(12):e114969

[28] Miao J, et al. Flavin-containing monooxygenase 3 as a potential player in diabetes-associated atherosclerosis. Nature Communications. 2015;**6**: 6498

[29] Xu R, Wang Q, Li L. A genome-wide systems analysis reveals strong link between colorectal cancer and trimethylamine N-oxide (TMAO), a gut microbial metabolite of dietary meat and fat. BMC Genomics. 2015;**16**(7):S4

[30] Bae S, et al. Relationship between plasma choline metabolites and risk of colorectal cancer in the Women's Health Initiative Observational Study (370.5). The FASEB Journal. 2014;**28**(1 Supplement):370.5

[31] Zeisel SH, et al. Choline, an essential nutrient for humans. The FASEB Journal. 1991; **5**(7):2093-2098

[32] Zeisel SH, et al. Concentrations of choline-containing compounds and betaine in common foods. Journal of Nutrition. 2003;**133**(5):1302-1307

[33] Craciun S, Balskus EP. Microbial conversion of choline to trimethylamine requires a glycyl radical enzyme. Proceedings of the National Academy of Sciences of the United States of America. 2012;**109**(52):21307-21312

[34] Koeth RA, et al. Intestinal microbiota metabolism of L-carnitine, a nutrient in red meat, promotes atherosclerosis. Nature Medicine. 2013;**19**(5):576-585

[35] Koeth RA, et al. gamma-Butyrobetaine is a proatherogenic intermediate in gut microbial metabolism of L-carnitine to TMAO. Cell Metabolism. 2014;**20**(5):799-812

[36] Zhu Y, et al. Carnitine metabolism to trimethylamine by an unusual Rieske-type oxygenase from human microbiota. Proceedings of the National Academy of Sciences of the United States of America. 2014;**111**(11):4268-4273

[37] Jameson E, et al. Metagenomic data-mining reveals contrasting microbial populations responsible for trimethylamine formation in human gut and marine ecosystems. Microbial Genomics. 2016;**2**(9):1-7

[38] Borrel G, et al. Genomics and metagenomics of trimethylamine-utilizing Archaea in the human gut microbiome. The ISME Journal. 2017. Advance online publication, 6 June 2017. DOI: 10.1038/ismej.2017.72

[39] Bennett BJ, et al. Trimethylamine-N-oxide, a metabolite associated with atherosclerosis, exhibits complex genetic and dietary regulation. Cell Metabolism. 2013;**17**(1):49-60

[40] Warrier M, et al. The TMAO-generating enzyme flavin monooxygenase 3 is a central regulator of cholesterol balance. Cell Reports. 2015;**10**(3):326-338

[41] Ayesh R, et al. The fish odour syndrome: Biochemical, familial, and clinical aspects. British Medical Journal. 1993;**307**(6905):655-657

[42] Mitchell SC, Smith RL. Trimethylaminuria: The fish malodor syndrome. Drug Metabolism and Disposition. 2001;**29**(4 Pt 2):517-521

[43] Al-Waiz M, et al. A genetic polymorphism of the N-oxidation of trimethylamine in humans. Clinical Pharmacology & Therapeutics. 1987;**42**(5):588-594

[44] Shephard EA, Treacy EP, Phillips IR. Clinical utility gene card for: Trimethylaminuria. European Journal of Human Genetics. 2012;**20**(3). DOI:10.1038/ejhg.2011.214

[45] Treacy EP, et al. Mutations of the flavin-containing monooxygenase gene (FMO3) cause trimethylaminuria, a defect in detoxication. Human Molecular Genetics. 1998;**7**(5):839-845

[46] Mackay RJ, et al. Trimethylaminuria: Causes and diagnosis of a socially distressing condition. The Clinical Biochemist Reviews. 2011;**32**(1):33-43

[47] Kris-Etherton PM, et al. Omega-3 fatty acids and cardiovascular disease: New recommendations from the American Heart Association. Arteriosclerosis Thrombosis and Vascular Biology. 2003;**23**(2):151-152

[48] Blusztajn JK. Choline, a vital amine. Science. 1998;**281**(5378):794-795

[49] Buchman AL, et al. Choline deficiency: A cause of hepatic steatosis during parenteral nutrition that can be reversed with intravenous choline supplementation. Hepatology. 1995;**22**(5):1399-1403

[50] Spencer MD, et al. Association between composition of the human gastrointestinal microbiome and development of fatty liver with choline deficiency. Gastroenterology. 2011;**140**(3):976-986

[51] De Filippis F, et al. High-level adherence to a Mediterranean diet beneficially impacts the gut microbiota and associated metabolome. Gut. DOI: 10.1136/gutjnl-2015-309957

[52] Chen ML, et al. Resveratrol attenuates trimethylamine-N-oxide (TMAO)-induced atherosclerosis by regulating TMAO synthesis and bile acid metabolism via remodeling of the gut microbiota. MBio. 2016;**7**(2):e02210–e02215

[53] Wang Z, et al. Non-lethal inhibition of gut microbial trimethylamine production for the treatment of atherosclerosis. Cell. 2015;**163**(7):1585-1595

[54] Jonsson AL, Bäckhed F. Drug the Bug! Cell. 2015;**163**(7):1565-1566

[55] Dambrova M, et al. Pharmacological effects of meldonium: Biochemical mechanisms and biomarkers of cardiometabolic activity. Pharmacological Research. 2016;**113**:771-780

[56] Dambrova M, et al. Meldonium decreases the diet-increased plasma levels of trimethylamine N-oxide, a metabolite associated with atherosclerosis. The Journal of Clinical Pharmacology. 2013;**53**(10):1095-1098

[57] Kuka J, et al. Suppression of intestinal microbiota-dependent production of pro-atherogenic trimethylamine N-oxide by shifting L-carnitine microbial degradation. Life Sciences. 2014;**117**(2):84-92

[58] Woese CR, Fox GE. Phylogenetic structure of the prokaryotic domain: the primary kingdoms. Proceedings of the National Academy of Sciences of the United States of America. 1977;**74**(11):5088-5090

[59] Koga Y, Morii H. Recent advances in structural research on ether lipids from archaea including comparative and physiological aspects. Bioscience, Biotechnology, and Biochemistry. 2005;**69**(11):2019-2034

[60] Spang A, et al. Complex archaea that bridge the gap between prokaryotes and eukaryotes. Nature. 2015;**521**(7551):173-179

[61] Thauer RK, et al. Methanogenic archaea: Ecologically relevant differences in energy conservation. Nature Reviews Microbiology. 2008;**6**(8):579-591

[62] Gaci N, et al. Archaea and the human gut: New beginning of an old story. World Journal of Gastroenterology. 2014;**20**(43):16062-16078

[63] Mihajlovski A, Alric M, Brugère J.-F. A putative new order of methanogenic Archaea inhabiting the human gut, as revealed by molecular analyses of the mcrA gene. Research in Microbiology. 2008;**159**(7-8):516-521

[64] Mihajlovski A, et al. Molecular evaluation of the human gut methanogenic archaeal microbiota reveals an age-associated increase of the diversity. Environmental Microbiology Reports. 2010;**2**(2):272-280

[65] Dridi B, et al. Methanomassiliicoccus luminyensis gen. nov., sp. nov., a methanogenic archaeon isolated from human faeces. International Journal of Systematic and Evolutionary Microbiology. 2012;**62**(Pt 8):1902-1907

[66] Iino T, et al. Candidatus Methanogranum caenicola: A novel methanogen from the anaerobic digested sludge, and proposal of Methanomassiliicoccaceae fam. nov. and *Methanomassiliicoccales* ord. nov., for a methanogenic lineage of the class Thermoplasmata. Microbes and Environments. 2013;**28**(2):244-250

[67] Borrel G, et al. Phylogenomic data support a seventh order of methylotrophic methanogens and provide insights into the evolution of methanogenesis. Genome Biology and Evolution. 2013;**5**(10):1769-1780

[68] Sollinger A, et al. Phylogenetic and genomic analysis of *Methanomassiliicoccales* in wetlands and animal intestinal tracts reveals clade-specific habitat preferences. FEMS Microbiology Ecology. 2016;**92**(1):pii: fiv149

[69] Paul K, et al. "Methanoplasmatales," Thermoplasmatales-related archaea in termite guts and other environments, are the seventh order of methanogens. Applied and Environmental Microbiology. 2012;**78**(23):8245-8253

[70] Henderson G, et al. Rumen microbial community composition varies with diet and host, but a core microbiome is found across a wide geographical range. Scientific Reports. 2015;**5**:14567

[71] Morgavi DP, et al. Rumen microbial communities influence metabolic phenotypes in lambs. Frontiers in Microbiology. 2015;**6**:1060

[72] Poulsen M, et al. Methylotrophic methanogenic Thermoplasmata implicated in reduced methane emissions from bovine rumen. Nature Communications. 2013;**4**:1428

[73] St-Pierre B, et al. Toward the identification of methanogenic archaeal groups as targets of methane mitigation in livestock animals. Frontiers in Microbiology. 2015;**6**:776

[74] Vanderhaeghen S, Lacroix C, Schwab C. Methanogen communities in stools of humans of different age and health status and co-occurrence with bacteria. FEMS Microbiology Letters. 2015;**362**(13):fnv092

[75] Borrel G, et al. Genome sequence of "Candidatus Methanomethylophilus alvus" Mx1201, a methanogenic archaeon from the human gut belonging to a seventh order of methanogens. Journal of Bacteriology. 2012;**194**(24):6944-6945

[76] Borrel G, et al. Comparative genomics highlights the unique biology of *Methanomassiliicoccales*, a Thermoplasmatales-related seventh order of methanogenic archaea that encodes pyrrolysine. BMC Genomics. 2014;**15**(1):679

[77] Lang K, et al. New mode of energy metabolism in the seventh order of methanogens as revealed by comparative genome analysis of "Candidatus methanoplasma termitum". Applied and Environmental Microbiology. 2015;**81**(4):1338-1352

[78] Becker KW, et al. Unusual butane- and pentanetriol-based tetraether lipids in methanomassiliicoccus luminyensis, a representative of the seventh order of methanogens. Applied and Environmental Microbiology. 2016;**82**(15):4505-4516

[79] Kroninger L, et al. Evidence for the involvement of two heterodisulfide reductases in the energy-conserving system of Methanomassiliicoccus luminyensis. The FEBS Journal. 2016;**283**(3):472-483

[80] Brugère JF, et al. Archaebiotics: Proposed therapeutic use of archaea to prevent trimethylaminuria and cardiovascular disease. Gut Microbes. 2014;**5**(1):5-10

[81] Gaston MA, Jiang R, Krzycki JA. Functional context, biosynthesis, and genetic encoding of pyrrolysine. Current Opinion in Microbiology. 2011;**14**(3):342-349

[82] Krzycki JA. The path of lysine to pyrrolysine. Current Opinion in Chemical Biology. 2013;**17**(4):619-625

[83] Longstaff DG, et al. A natural genetic code expansion cassette enables transmissible biosynthesis and genetic encoding of pyrrolysine. Proceedings of the National Academy of Sciences of the United States of America. 2007;**104**(3):1021-1026

[84] Borrel G, et al. Genome sequence of "Candidatus Methanomassiliicoccus intestinalis" issoire-Mx1, a third thermoplasmatales-related methanogenic archaeon from human feces. Genome Announcements. 2013;**1**(4):e00453-13

[85] Claesson MJ, et al. Gut microbiota composition correlates with diet and health in the elderly. Nature. 2012;**488**(7410):178-184

[86] O'Toole PW, Jeffery IB. Gut microbiota and aging. Science. 2015;**350**(6265):1214-1215

[87] Chaudhary PP, et al. Molecular methods for studying methanogens of the human gastrointestinal tract: Current status and future directions. Applied Microbiology and Biotechnology. 2015;**99**(14):5801-5815

[88] Clemente JC, et al. The microbiome of uncontacted Amerindians. Science Advances. 2015;**1**(3):e1500183

[89] Liu DM, et al. The probiotic role of Lactobacillus plantarum in reducing risks associated with cardiovascular disease. International Journal of Food Science & Technology. 2017;**52**(1):127-136

[90] Feria-Gervasio D, et al. In vitro maintenance of a human proximal colon microbiota using the continuous fermentation system P-ECSIM. Applied Microbiology and Biotechnology. 2011;**91**(5):1425-1433

[91] Feria-Gervasio D, et al. Three-stage continuous culture system with a self-generated anaerobia to study the regionalized metabolism of the human gut microbiota. Journal of Microbiological Methods. 2014;**96**:111-118

[92] Tottey W, et al. In-vitro model for studying methanogens in human gut microbiota. Anaerobe. 2015;**34**:50-52

[93] Gorlas A, et al. Complete genome sequence of *Methanomassiliicoccus luminyensis*, the largest genome of a human-associated Archaea species. Journal of bacteriology.**194**(17): 4745-4745

[94] Kelly WJ, et al. Complete genome sequence of methanogenic archaeon ISO4-G1, a member of the *Methanomassiliicoccales,* isolated from a sheep rumen. Genome announcements; **4**(2):e00221-e00216

[95] Li Y, et al. The complete genome sequence of the methanogenic archaeon ISO4-H5 provides insights into the methylotrophic lifestyle of a ruminal representative of the Methanomassiliicoccales. Standards in Genomic Sciences;**11**(1):59

[96] Noel SJ, et al. Draft genome sequence of "Candidatus Methanomethylophilus" sp. 1R26, enriched from bovine rumen, a methanogenic archaeon belonging to the Methano massiliicoccales order. Genome announcements;**4**(1):e01734-15

Chapter 4

Biocompounds from Haloarchaea and Their Uses in Biotechnology

Javier Torregrosa-Crespo, Carmen Pire Galiana and
Rosa María Martínez-Espinosa

Additional information is available at the end of the chapter

http://dx.doi.org/10.5772/intechopen.69944

Abstract

New advances in the understanding of haloarchaea physiology, metabolism, biochemistry, and molecular biology show that these kinds of microorganisms produce several compounds in response to the extreme conditions of their ecosystems. Thus, the complete metabolic and genetic machineries are fully adapted to nutrient starvation, high sun radiation, and high ionic strength. Due to these adaptations, some of the primary and secondary metabolites produced by haloarchaea are of high interest in terms of potential biotechnological uses. The principal goal of the chapter is to present a review about the main characteristics of these biocompounds and their potential uses in biomedicine, pharmacy, and industry.

Keywords: biotechnology, carotenoids, enzymes, haloarchaea, natural pigments, polyhydroxyalkanoates

1. Introduction

Hypersaline environments such as hypersaline lakes, soils, springs, solar salterns, and rock salt deposits are widely distributed around the world. Organisms inhabiting these ecosystems are characterized by their high salt tolerance/requirements [1]. The organisms living under these conditions are usually termed "halotolerants/halophiles/halophilic organisms." The term "halophilic" means "salt-loving." The most widely used definitions distinguish different categories:

(i) Extreme halophiles: growing best in media containing 2.5–5.2 M salt;

(ii) Borderline extreme halophiles: growing best in media containing 1.5–4.0 M salt;

(iii) Moderate halophiles: growing best in media containing 0.5–2.5 M salt; and

(iv) Halotolerant microorganisms: salt is not an absolute requirement for their growth, but they can grow even in the presence of very high salt concentrations (considered extremely halotolerant if the growth range extends above 2.5 M salt).

These kinds of definitions have proved valuable in the classification of microorganisms based on their relationship to salt [2–5].

Halophilic microorganisms can be found in all three domains of life (Archaea, Bacteria, and Eukarya). However, those that require high salt concentrations for optimal growth (2–4 M NaCl) are mainly archaea grouped into the families *Halobacteriaceae* and *Haloferacaceae*, phylum Euryarchaeota [6]. They constitute the main populations in highly salty environments like marshes or salty ponds, where NaCl is obtained for human consumption [7].

Halophilic archaea (haloarchaea) are mostly aerobic, although some species can grow anaerobically using nitrate as the final electron acceptor (denitrification) [8]. Most of the species are generally red-pigmented. To be alive under these extreme conditions (low water availability, high sun radiation, nutrient starvation, and high ionic strength), halophilic microbes show different metabolic adaptations. Some of the main adaptations are:

(i) Cells accumulate high KCl intracellular concentrations or some osmolytes such as 2-sulfotrehalose to deal with high ionic strength [9]. This "salt-in" strategy is mainly used by haloarchaea and it requires the adaptation of the intracellular enzymatic machinery, as proteins should maintain their proper conformation and activity at near-saturating salt concentrations [1, 3, 4].

(ii) Amino acidic residues predominate on halophilic proteins' surface. Thus, proteins become stable and active within cytoplasms containing high KCl concentrations. Consequently, the proteome of such microorganisms is highly acidic, and most proteins denature when they are suspended in low salt concentration [1, 3, 4].

(iii) Cellular bilayers have different composition and structure [10].

(iv) Genomes from halophilic microorganisms contain significant amount of salt resistance genes [11].

Due to these adaptations, some of the primary and secondary metabolites produced by haloarchaea are of high interest in biotechnology. Thus, several biocompounds such as enzymes [12], carotenoids [13], PHAs/PHBs [14], and halocins (bacteriocin-like peptides) [15] have focused the attention of many researchers around the world. Many of the studies on these subjects were published between the 1990s and the first decade of the current century. However, large-scale industrial applications from archaeal cultures are yet to come. Several technical difficulties must be addressed in the near future to make possible efficient large-scale biotechnological applications using archaea. In that sense, aspects related to fermenter corrosion, for instance, should be properly analyzed.

http://dx.doi.org/10.5772/intechopen.69944

This work summarizes what has been described so far about biocompounds produced by haloarchaea (mainly enzymes, pigments, and bioplastics), their production at large scale, as well as the potential uses of these biocompounds in biotechnology, biomedicine, pharmacy, and industry.

2. Carotenoids

2.1. Carotenoids: definition, classification, and metabolism

Natural pigments are widespread in all organisms. They provide attractive colors and play basic biological roles in the development of organisms [16]. Among natural pigments, carotenoids are of high interest due to their biotechnological applications and their potential beneficial effects on human health [17–19]. These compounds are the second most abundant naturally occurring pigments in nature ranging from colorless to yellow, orange, and red [20, 21]. The production of these pigments has been described in plants and some microorganisms such as algae, cyanobacteria, yeast, and fungi [22, 23]. From a chemical point of view, carotenoids are hydrophobic compounds, which essentially consist of a C_{40} hydrocarbon backbone in the case of carotenes (i.e., they contain 40 carbon atoms in eight isoprene residues), often modified by various oxygen-containing functional groups to produce cyclic or acyclicxanthophylls. Thus, all carotenoids are characterized by the following common features: long-conjugated chain of double bond and a near-bilateral symmetry around the central double bond [24]. This chain may be terminated by cyclic groups (rings), and it can be complemented with oxygen-containing functional groups [25].

Carotenoids can be classified into different groups using different criteria. Considering the chemical structure and the oxygen presence, two types can be distinguished: carotenes or carotenoid hydrocarbons, composed of carbon and hydrogen only; and xanthophylls or oxygenated carotenoids, which are oxygenated and may contain epoxy, carbonyl, hydroxyl, methoxy, or carboxylic acid functional groups [26]. Lycopene and β-carotene are examples of carotene carotenoids and lutein, canthaxanthin, zeaxanthin, violaxanthin, capsorubin and astaxanthin are xanthopyll carotenoids [27].

These natural pigments are derived from the general isoprenoid biosynthetic pathway, along with a variety of other important natural substances such as steroids and gibberellic acid. In this pathway, mevalonic acid is the starting product which is further transformed into a phosphorylated isoprene upon phosphorylation; this isoprene subsequently polymerizes. During polymerization, the number and position of the double bonds are fixed. The conversion of two molecules of geranylgeranyl pyrophosphate (GGPP) to phytoene, a compound common to all C_{40} carotenogenic organisms, constitutes the first reaction unique to the carotenoid branch of isoprenoid metabolism. From this step, slightly different reactions can be found in different organisms [13].

The synthesis and degradation of carotenes and xanthophylls, the regulation of carotenogenesis, as well as the role of these compounds, have been very well described in plants [20] and mammals [28]. Animals are not able to synthesize carotenoids *de novo*, and consequently, they are acquired through diet. In most of the organisms, carotenoids show powerful antioxidant properties, which directly emerge from their molecular structure [13].

2.2. Carotenoids produced by haloarchaea

Bibliography about carotenoids of extremophile microorganisms is scarce as compared to all information available from other organisms [29]. Nevertheless, it has been demonstrated that most members of the families *Haloferacaceae* and *Halobacteriaceae* can synthesize C_{50} carotenoids, including bacterioruberin (as the most abundant C_{50} in most of the analyzed haloarchaeal species) and its precursors (2-isopentenyl-3,4-dehydrorhodopin (IDR), bisanhydrobacterioruberin (BABR), and monoanhydrobacterioruberin (MABR)) [30, 31]. Bacterioruberin has a rather different molecular structure. It has a primary conjugated isoprenoid chain length of 13 C=C units with no subsidiary conjugation arising from terminal groups, which contain four —OH group functionalities only (**Figure 1**) [32].

Several other derivatives have been found in minor amounts: 3,4-dehidromonoanhydrobacterioruberin, haloxanthin (which is a derivative of the previous one containing a peroxide end group), and 3,4-epoxymonoanhydrobacterioruberin, identified in *Haloferax volcanii* [33]. Carotenoids such as phytoene, lycopene, and β-carotene are also produced by these species but at lower concentration. Usually, these carotenoids are in the cell membranes, and they provide color to the colonies when haloarchaea cells grow on solid media or sustain the red color shown by salted coastal ponds (mainly in summer).

Thanks to bacterioruberin and its derivatives, haloarchaeal cells are protected against UV sun radiations. They are also involved in the reinforcement of the cell membrane, and they can be part of the rhodopsin complexes (light-driven proton pump highly important for haloarchaea cells to obtain energy) [13].

The effect of several chemical compounds on the C_{50} carotenoids biosynthesis was first described from *Halobacterium cutirubrum* (*Halobacteriaceae* family) [31]. Few years later, it was described that bacterioruberin is in general synthesized from other C_{50} carotenoids, such as isopentenyldehydrorhodopin, bisanhydrobacterioruberin, and monoanhydrobacterioruberin [21]. The synthesis is induced by (i) low oxygen tension and high light intensity [34, 35]; (ii) osmotic stress [36]; and (iii) the presence of different compounds such as aniline (**Figure 1**) [37]. However, this general pattern has some exceptions, for example *Haloquadratum walsbyi*:

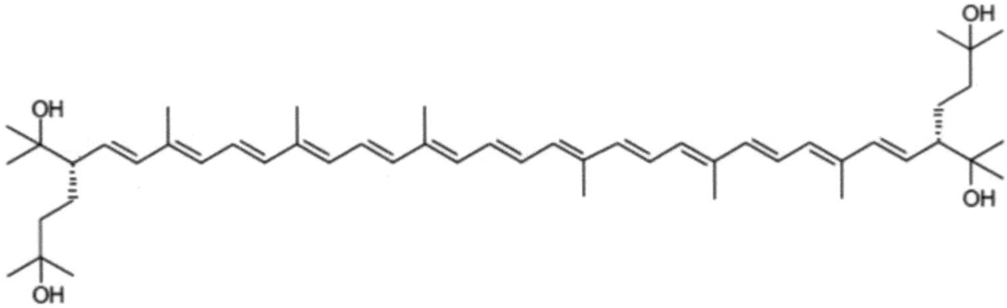

Figure 1. Chemical structure of bacterioruberin.

cells grown under osmotic stress did not experience changes in terms of either membrane lipid content or carotenoid production [38]. Composition of the total carotenoid fraction in haloarchaeal cells can also vary based on the nutritive factors within the culture media [39], the light intensity, oxygen tension, NaCl concentration [39, 40], and other physical-chemical parameters such as the pH value of the culture media.

2.3. Applications and prospects

Few studies stated that some haloarchaeal species (wild-type strains) produce significant concentrations of carotenoids, which are marked highly demanding [13]. Besides, carotenoid production by haloarchaea can be improved by genetic modification or even by modifying several cultivation aspects such as nutrition, growth pH, or temperature.

There are no studies on the potential benefits of the carotenoids produced by haloarchaea on human health reported in the scientific literature up to now. However, there are some patents in which the potential use of haloarchaeal carotenoids in biomedicine and biotechnology has been tested [13]. More efforts should be made not only to explore biotechnological uses of haloarchaeal carotenoids at large scale, but also to open marks related to carotenoid synthesis and degradation in haloarchaea. This knowledge will promote progress in the field of carotenoid metabolic engineering in these microbes, and it will contribute to evaluating the potential use of haloarchaea as sources for carotenoids production at large scale.

3. Enzymes

Enzymes from halophilic archaea are active and stable at high salinity conditions which are environments generally adverse to other enzymes. Compared to non-halophilic enzymes, they are characterized by a relatively higher usage of acidic residues, a low frequency of lysine, and a high occurrence of amino acids with a low hydrophobic character. This composition makes the proteins' surface acidic with a decrease in hydrophobic patches [41, 42]. Analysis of *Haloferax mediterranei* glucose dehydrogenase structure also reveals an absence of very mobile side chains on the surface that allow the formation of a highly ordered multilayered solvation shell. This feature is necessary under the water-limited conditions characterizing salty environments [42]. Halophilic enzymes present thermophilic character too; consequently, they are stable in a broad range of temperatures. Haloarchaea may endure high temperatures in their natural environment, and halophilic protein need to be not only soluble at high salt concentrations but thermostable as well [43, 44].

These unique characteristics make halophilic enzymes very attractive for biotechnological applications. They are also active and stable in media with low water activity as in the presence of organic solvents [45, 46], even at low salt concentrations if they are encapsulated in reverse micelles. Under these conditions, halophilic enzymes could be used in biotechnological applications in non-aqueous media [47, 48].

Many enzymes from haloarchaea with potential interest, such as glycosyl hydrolases, proteases, lipases, and esterases, have been characterized, but no large-scale applications have been reported yet. In this section, the main features characterizing haloarchaeal enzymes suitable to be used for biotechnological applications are described:

3.1. Glycosyl hydrolases

Glycosyl hydrolases are enzymes capable of hydrolyzing glucosidic bonds between carbohydrates. They are classified into 108 families based on amino acid similarities [49]. Among them, starch-hydrolyzing enzymes are of special interest since their substrate has attracted industrial attention in versatile processes, essentially in the food and detergent industries [50]. Hydrolysis of starch demands the coordinated activity of several enzymes. Most of the known starch-modifying enzymes can be found in the glycosyl hydrolase family 13 which includes α-amylases, pullulanases, α-1,6-glucosidases, branching enzymes, maltogenic amylases, neopullulanases, and cyclodextrinases [51].

Some halophilic amylases from Archaea have been characterized [51–55]. Most of them retain their activity at high temperatures. For example, the haloarchaeon *H. mediterranei* secretes an α-amylase showing optimum temperature between 50 and 60°C, but it retains 65% of the maximum activity at 80°C [55]. *H. mediterranei* also has a monomeric extracellular cyclodextrin glycosyltransferase working optimally at 55°C and 1.5 M NaCl, but it is active even at low salt concentrations as 0.5 M NaCl (retaining 65% of its activity) [56]. Cyclodextrins are interesting molecules because of their ability to form inclusion complexes with organic molecules, increasing their solubility in aqueous solutions.

As mentioned earlier, due to the low water activity in the environments inhabited by haloarchaea, many of their enzymes are functional in organic and hydrophobic solvents. For example, the amylase of *Haloarcula* sp. works optimally at 4.3 M salt and 50°C, but the enzyme does not lose its activity at low salt concentrations. Even in the absence of NaCl, it maintains more than 30% activity. The enzyme is also stable in benzene, toluene, and chloroform, showing its potential as a good candidate for industrial applications [45].

3.2. Cellulases and chitinases

Halophilic cellulases have recently generated interest by their application in biofuel production. Plant biomass, which is the starting material, consists mainly of cellulose, hemicellulose, and lignin. Especially the latter one is highly resistant to biodegradation processes, which involves the use of harsh pre-treatments (high temperatures and extreme pH conditions). Alkali pre-treatments can be done using alkaline salts, resulting in pH and salt concentrations like those found in alkaline saline lakes. Besides, ionic liquids (ILs) can efficiently solubilize cellulose, hemicellulose, and lignin under moderate temperatures. Thus, enzymes from halophilic archaea are good candidates to resist the extreme conditions of these processes [57].

Zhang et al. have identified and characterized a halophilic cellulase (Hu-CBH1) from the halophilic archaeon *Halorhabdus utahensis* [57], which is a heat-tolerant haloalkaliphilic enzyme. It is active in salt concentrations up to 5 M NaCl, pH 11.5, and high levels of ILs. These results indicate that enzymes isolated from hypersaline environments are strong candidates for the development of IL-tolerant enzymes and cocktails capable of releasing monomeric sugars from IL-pre-treated biomass efficiently [57].

Two *Haloarcula* strains with cellulolytic activity were isolated from the saline soil of Yuncheng Salt Lake, China [58, 59]. Crude cellulase of strain LLSG7 was a multicomponent enzyme system, which showed endoglucanase, cellobiohydrolase, and β-glucosidase activities [59]. The cellulase secreted by strain G10 was an endoglucanase suitable for soluble cellulose degradation [58]. Both were highly active and stable over broad ranges of temperature, pH, and NaCl concentrations, and they displayed remarkable stability in the presence of non-polar organic solvents. The crude cellulase of strain LLSG7 was applied to hydrolyze alkali-pre-treated rice straw, and the enzymatic hydrolysate was used as the substrate for bioethanol fermentation by *Saccharomyces cerevisiae*. The yield of bioethanol obtained suggested it might potentially be used for its production [59].

Although several cellulases had been isolated previously, Sorokin and co-workers demonstrated for the first time that extremely halophilic archaea can grow in insoluble chitin and cellulose as a sole growth substrate in salt-saturated mineral media, indicating that euryarchaea participate in aerobic mineralization of recalcitrant organic polymers in environments saturated with salts [60].

As cellulases, chitinolytic enzymes have wide-ranging applications, such as the preparation of chitooligosaccharides and N-acetylglucosamines used in the pharmaceutical industry [61]. Chitinases are glycosyl hydrolases that catalyze the hydrolytic degradation of the β-1,4-glycosidic bonds present in chitin. It is one of the most abundant polysaccharides in nature besides cellulose and starch. The main natural chitin sources are the shells of crustaceans, insect exoskeletons, and fungal cell walls. A chitinolytic extremozyme from the halophilic archaeon *Halobacterium salinarum* showed the highest activity in the presence of 1.5 M NaCl, even retaining 20% of its activity in the absence of salt. It is an exo-acting enzyme with potential interest regarding the biodegradation of chitin waste or its bioconversion into biologically active products.

Hou et al. have identified the genes and enzymes involved in chitin catabolism in *H. mediterranei*, being the first time that this process has been described in haloarchaea. The study demonstrates that *H. mediterranei* can use colloidal or powdered chitin for both cell growth and poly(3-hydroxybutyrate-co-3-hydroxyvalerate) (PHBV) biosynthesis (see Section 4), suggesting the potential of this strain for conversion of chitin into valuable bioplastics [62].

3.3. Proteases

Proteolytic enzymes are used to produce pharmaceuticals, foods, detergents, leather, silk, and agrochemical products. In terms of production, proteases represent the heart of the global market for enzymes [63].

Proteases from halophilic microorganisms have been reviewed recently [64]. In general terms, haloarchaeal proteases show optimum activity at high salt concentration, although some of them can be stable and active at lower concentrations. The extracellular endopeptidase from *Halobacterium halobium* hydrolyzes polypeptides and oligopeptides with specificity for hydrophobic amino acids, especially proline [65]. The enzyme exhibits azocasein activity at low salt concentrations. This endopeptidase could be an important tool to be used in the food processing industry as well as in biomedical applications to produce peptides [65, 66].

Kim and Dordick studied the stability of a protease from *H. halobium* in different aqueous/organic solvent mixtures, and they observed that it correlates strongly with the salting-out ability of the solvent [46]. They concluded that solvents which act to increase the apparent hydrophobicity of the enzyme's core stabilize it in the same way as salting-out salts [46]. Finally, the p-nitrophenylphosphate phosphatase from *H. salinarum* was dissolved in an organic medium by creating a reverse micellar system at very low salt concentration and, under these conditions, the enzyme was active and stable [67]. The possibility of using these enzymes in hydrophobic medium increases the potential biotechnological applications.

3.4. Esterases and lipases

Esterases and lipases hydrolyze ester bonds between a fatty acid moiety and an esterified conjugate, such as a glycerol or phosphate. Lipases preferentially hydrolyze triglycerides composed of long-chain fatty acids while esterases usually hydrolyze water-soluble esters, including short-chain fatty acid triglycerides. Both enzymes have applications in food modification, detergent formulation, cosmetic, pharmaceutical, leather, textile, paper industries, biodiesel and biopolymer production, or pre-treatment of lipid-rich wastewaters [68]. These applications often require aggressive reaction conditions: high temperatures to sustain biocatalysis, organic solvents as part of the reaction mixtures, or presence of high salt concentration. Thus, extremophilic enzymes (especially halophilic enzymes) can be a very interesting option. The biotechnological applications of halophilic lipases and thioesterases have been reviewed recently [69]. Bhatnagar et al. isolated 54 Halobacteria from a salt lake in the Algerian Sahara and screened 35 of these strains [70]. Among them, strain TC6 (belonging to the *Natronococcus* genus) was selected for further study. It contains an extracellular lipase that was optimally active at 4 M NaCl, pH 7, and 50°C, and it was more active against the substrate p-nitrophenyl palmitate (C16). The enzyme hydrolyzed olive oil, indicating the presence of a true lipase, being the first one reported in archaea [71]. After that, a total of 118 halophilic archaeal strains were screened for lipolytic activity. Five isolates were selected and further characterized, indicating the presence of salt-dependent and temperature-tolerant lipolytic enzymes [72]. Camacho et al. studied the production of esterase and lipase in *Haloarcula marismortui* [73]: they observed high production rates of intracellular esterase and lipase using p-nitrophenyl valerate and p-nitrophenyl laurate, respectively. Two different esterases were detected as active enzymes at 0.5 and 5 M NaCl. Interestingly, in the absence of salt, esterase retained 50% of residual activity [73].

Moreover, Müller-Santos et al. cloned and overexpressed the *lipC* gene from *H. marismortui* [74]. The recombinant protein was purified and biochemically characterized. The enzyme exhibited preference for short-chain fatty acids and monoesters, and its optimum activity was observed in the presence of 3 M KCl while no activity was detected in the absence of salts.

http://dx.doi.org/10.5772/intechopen.69944

An area of interest for the application of halophilic lipases is biofuel production. With this aim, a lipase from a haloarchaeal strain G41 was purified to homogeneity and characterized [75]. The enzyme displayed high stability and activity in the presence of hydrophobic organic solvents and showed preference toward long-chain substrates, which makes the enzyme suitable for biofuel production. The free and immobilized lipase from strain G41 was applied for biodiesel production, and 80.5 and 89.2% of yields were achieved, respectively [75]. This study demonstrated the feasibility of using lipases from halophilic archaea for biodiesel production.

4. Polyhydroxyalkanoates (PHAs)

4.1. Polyhydroxyalkanoates: definition, classification, and biosynthesis

PHAs are polyesters composed of hydroxy fatty acids, synthesized and stored as insoluble inclusions in the cytoplasm [76]. They serve as intracellular storage material of carbon source and energy. PHAs are produced in the stationary phase of growth, when the medium is deficient in some essential nutrients but a carbon source is available in excess. When it is running out, PHAs are depolymerized, and their degradation products are used for growth [77].

There is a wide variety of types of PHAs, depending on different aspects such as the microorganism strain, the growth conditions, or the carbon source used. To date, over 150 structural variations have been reported [78, 79]. There are different ways to classify these biopolymers: on the one hand, depending upon the number of carbon atoms in the monomers, PHAs are classified into two distinct groups [77, 79]: scl-PHAs (short-chain length PHAs), whose monomers consist of 3–5 carbon atoms, and mcl-PHAs (medium chain length PHAs), composed of monomers having 6–14 carbon atoms; on the other hand, PHAs can be classified depending on the type of monomers that form them [78, 79]: the homopolymers, made of identical monomers, include PHB (poly-3-hydroxybutyrate), P3HP (poly-3-hydroxypropionate), P4HB (poly-4-hydroxybutyrate), PTE (polythioester), PLA (polylactic acid), and PHV(polyhydroxyvalerate), among others; copolymers (also called heteropolymers), derived from more than one species of monomer like PHBV (polyhydroxybutyrate-valerate). In addition, the variety of PHAs is higher considering more aspects, such as the structure of their side chains (saturated or not) and the presence of aromatic or halogenated groups in their monomers [77].

PHAs are synthesized by four natural pathways [78]: pathway I, that converts sugar to acetyl-CoA, acetoacetyl-CoA to 3-hydroxybutyryl-CoA which is polymerized to PHB; pathway II, that begins from fatty acids to produce R-3-hydroxyacyl-CoA monomers for PHA synthesis via β-oxidation cycle; pathway III, that converts acetyl-CoA, malonyl-CoA to 3-ketoacyl-ACP into R-3-hydroxyacyl-CoA monomers; pathway IV converts butyric acid to S-3-hydroxybutyryl-CoA, then to acetyl-CoA to form PHA monomers.

All these metabolic pathways end with monomer polymerization to produce PHAs. The enzymes responsible for this reaction are PHA synthases. Therefore, it is considered that the key enzymes for PHA production are the polyester synthases [76, 78, 80]. In the Bacteria domain, where these kind of proteins have been studied extensively, they are divided into four classes depending on the subunit composition and their substrate [76, 77, 80].

Class I and II are PHA synthases that consist of only one type of subunit (PhaC) with molecular masses between 61 and 73 kDa [80]. The difference lies in the substrate specificity: while class I PHA synthases utilize CoA thioesters of various 3-hydroxy fatty acids comprising 3–5 carbon atoms, class II PHA synthases use CoA thioesters of 3-hydroxy fatty acids with 6–14 carbon atoms [76, 80].

The PHA synthases of class III consist of two subunits, PhaC and PhaE, both with similar molecular weight (around 40 kDa). These kinds of enzymes prefer as substrate CoA thioesters of 3-hydroxy fatty acids with three to five carbon atoms [80].

Class IV PHA synthases are like class III but the PhaE subunit is replaced by PhaR (with molecular mass around 20 kDa). They use 3-hydroxy fatty acids with three to five carbon atoms as substrate [80, 81].

4.2. Haloarchaea as polyhydroxyalkanoate producers

Polyhydroxyalkanoates have been extensively studied in the Bacteria domain, from biochemical and molecular biology points of view. However, in the Archaea domain, knowledge is more limited, although haloarchaea seem to be good models to produce these biopolymers. PHAs have been found in strains belonging to the genera *Haloferax, Haloarcula, Natrialba, Haloterrigena, Halococcus, Haloquadratum, Halorubrum, Natronobacterium, Natronococcus*, and *Halobacterium* [76].

The archaeal PHA synthases are composed of two subunits, PhaE and PhaC, that are homologous to the class III PHA synthases from bacteria with only two differences: first, they present a longer C-terminal extension in the PhaC subunit; second, the PhaE subunit lacks the hydrophobic and amphiphilic amino acids for granule association and it is much smaller than its bacterial counterpart [82, 83]. All these evidences make that haloarchaea PHA synthases are classified as PHA synthases of class III but in a differentiated subgroup [83].

The advantages of using haloarchaea to produce PHAs are numerous: first, these microorganisms have simple growth requirements; second, the presence of high salt concentrations in their growth media prevents any kind of contamination from other organisms, so the requirements for sterile conditions can be reduced [14, 84]; moreover, the biopolymers obtained can be easily recovered by osmotic shock of cells using media with low salinity or even distilled water [14], so it is not necessary to use any solvents to extract them.

Different haloarchaea strains have been tested as potential PHA producers using numerous carbon sources, fermentation techniques, and downstream steps. The two most studied genera are probably *Haloarcula* and *Haloferax*. Within the genus *Haloarcula, Haloarcula* sp. IRU1 has been the most productive strain, obtaining PHB as biopolymer with a yield of 63% (w/w) of cell dry weight (CDW). Glucose was used as carbon source [85]. Other *Haloarcula* strains tested were *H. marismortui* and *Haloarcula hispanica*, but the yields obtained were 21 and 2.4% (w/w) CDW, respectively [82, 86].

With respect to the *Haloferax* genus, *H. volcanii* and *Haloferax gibbonsii* showed growth in the presence of glucose and yeast extract as carbon and nitrogen sources, producing PHB as biopolymer with yields of 7 and 1.2% (w/w) CDW [86]. However, *H. mediterranei* is probably the best-studied strain in terms of producing PHAs [84, 87, 88]. Besides the advantages that the haloarchaea present to produce PHAs, *H. mediterranei* has a relatively high growth rate and exhibits high production of the copolymer PHBHV instead of PHB [14].

PHBHV is a copolymer form of 3-hydroxybutyrate (3HB) and 3-hydroxyvalerate (3HV). It presents improved properties compared to the homopolymer PHB, which is a brittle plastic that considerably limits its application [84]. Instead, PHBHV has similar properties to polypropylene: high impact resistance, toughness, and flexibility [14].

The main studies using *H. mediterranei* as model organism have been focused on the improvement of the accumulation of PHBHV and the reduction of the costs of production. Cheap carbon sources such as glycerol [89, 90], rice bran [91], rice-based ethanol stillage [92], cheese whey [93], and olive mill wastewater (the effluent of the olive oil industry) have been tested using multistage processes [94, 95] or only one-stage process (**Table 1**) [14].

	Olive mill wastewater [14]	**Hydrolyzed cheese whey [93]**	**Rice-based ethanol stillage [92]**	**Crude glycerol phase from biodiesel production [90]**	**Crude glycerol phase from biodiesel production and γ-butyrolactone [90]**	**Extruded rice bran and starch [91]**
Cultivation mode	Batch shake flasks	Batch reactor	Batch shake flasks	Fed-batch reactor	Fed-batch reactor	Fed-batch reactor
Biopolymer						
Type of biopolymer	PHBHV	PHBHV	PHBHV	PHBHV	PHBHV	PHBHV
3-HV content/ PHBHV (mol %)	6.5	1.5	15.4	10	11–12	–
Yield						
Protein (g L^{-1})	10	7.54	–	5.5	5.6	65.1
PHA concentration (g L^{-1})	0.2	7.92	16.42	16.2	11.11	77.8
PHA/CDM (%)	43	53	71	–	–	55.6

Table 1. Cultivation mode, type of biopolymer produced, and maximum polymer yields for cultivations of *H. mediterranei* in different waste sources.

4.3. Applications and prospects

PHAs have received considerable attention because of their industrial applications as biodegradable and biocompatible polymers [84]. These exhibit similarities with the conventional petrochemical-derived plastics, but they can be biodegradable in different environments [76]. The fields in which PHAs can be applied are varied: in the packaging industry, where they can compete with nondegradable polymers in the production of bottles and containers [96–98]; in biomedicine, as osteosynthetic materials, sutures, and wound dressing due to PHB's compatibility with the blood and tissues of mammals [98]; and in pharmaceutical applications for the controlled release of medicines [84].

Nowadays, there are numerous important companies that develop and commercialize different types of PHAs such as Biomer (Germany), PHB Industrial (Brazil), Bio-on (Italy) or Telles LLC (USA), which sell these biopolymers under the commercial name Metabolix.

In spite of all the advantages that these biopolymers present, their production on a large scale is still complicated: first, the PHAs production cost is still high (7–10 Euros/kilogram) [98]; second, petroleum, as a raw material for conventional plastics, has not increased its price dramatically in the last few years [99]; third, PHA processing is more difficult than petrochemical plastics due to their slow crystallization processes [100]; fourth, PHAs do not have consistent structures and properties compared to conventional plastics [99]. Therefore, nowadays PHAs are not products that can compete with plastics derived from the petrochemical industry yet.

The future objectives for PHA production remain the same as when these biopolymers were discovered: improving the productivity and reducing their costs, innovating in the use of waste carbon sources, improving genetically the microbial strains used, and using shorter downstream steps. In this sense, haloarchaea can be good models for the achievement of these objectives since their nutritional requirements are low and the processes to obtain these biopolymers are easier than in many bacterial species.

5. Conclusions

Haloarchaea (wild-type strains) can produce high concentrations of biocompounds that are of high interest for biotechnological purposes. Consequently, these microorganisms reveal new natural sources from which enzymes, pigments, and other secondary metabolites can be produced. Among other biocompounds of interest, halocins are of special relevance. These are bacteriocin-like substances (antibiotics) capable of killing sensitive halobacterial cells by affecting the bioenergetic steady state across the membrane [101, 102]. Potential uses of these specific antibiotics in biotechnology, pharmacy, and biomedicine produced by haloarchaea remain unexplored. The cells themselves are also promising systems to explore other uses such as biosensors or soil/water bioremediation strategies [8, 103]. Nevertheless, great effort must be made in the near future to scale-up the engineering tools required to produce biocompounds from haloarchaea at high concentrations or to use haloarchaeal whole cells for biotechnological purposes at large scale.

Acknowledgements

Most of the recent studies on enzymes and carotenoids from haloarchaea carried out in our laboratory have been supported by several grants from MINECO and Generalitat Valenciana (Spain). MINECO: CTM2013-43147-R; Generalitat Valenciana: APE/2016/045; ACIF/2016/077.

Author details

Javier Torregrosa-Crespo, Carmen Pire Galiana and Rosa María Martínez-Espinosa*

*Address all correspondence to: rosa.martinez@ua.es

Departamento de Agroquímica y Bioquímica, Facultad de Ciencias, Universidad de Alicante, Alicante, Spain

References

[1] Oren A. Microbial life at high salt concentrations: Phylogenetic and metabolic diversity. Saline Systems. 2008;**4**(2):1-13

[2] Kushner DJ. Life in high salt and solute concentrations. In: Kushner DJ, editor. Microbial Life in Extreme Environments. Academic Press; London. 1978. pp. 317-368

[3] Oren A. Halophilic Microorganisms and their Environments. Dordrecht: Kluwer Scientific Publishers; 2002

[4] Oren A. Life at high salt concentrations. In: Dworkin M, Falkow S, Rosenberg E, Schleifer KH, Stackebrandt E, editors. The Prokaryotes, A Handbook on the Biology of Bacteria: Ecophysiology and Biochemistry. Springer; New York. 2006. pp. 263-282

[5] Ventosa A, Nieto JJ, Oren A. Biology of aerobic moderately halophilic bacteria. Microbiology and Molecular Biology Reviews. 1998;**62**(2):504-544

[6] Gupta RS, Naushad S, Fabros R, et al. A phylogenomic reappraisal of family-level divisions within the class Halobacteria: Proposal to divide the order *Halobacteriales* into the families *Halobacteriaceae, Haloarculaceae* fam. nov., and *Halococcaceae* fam. nov., and the order *Haloferacales* into the families, *Haloferacaceae* and *Halorubraceae* famnov. Antonie Van Leeuwenhoek. 2016;**109**:565-587. DOI: 10.1007/s10482-016-0660-2

[7] Oren A. Life at high salt concentrations, intracellular KCl concentrations, and acidic proteomes. Frontiers in Microbiology. 2013;**4**:315

[8] Torregrosa-Crespo J, Martínez-Espinosa RM, Esclapez J, Bautista V, Pire C, Camacho M, Richardson DJ, Bonete MJ. Anaerobic metabolism in *Haloferax* genus: Denitrification as case of study. Advances in Microbial Physiology. 2016;**68**:41-85. DOI: 10.1016/bs.ampbs.2016.02.001

[9] Desmarais D, Jablonski PE, Fedarko NS, et al. 2-Sulfotrehalose, a novel osmolyte in haloalkaliphilic archaea. Journal of Bacteriology. 1997;**179**:3146-3153

[10] Mesbah NM, Wiegel J. Life under multiple extreme conditions: Diversity and physiology of the halophilic alkalithermophiles. Applied Environmental Microbiology. 2012;**78**:4074-4082

[11] Mirete S, Mora-Ruiz MR, Lamprecht-Grandío M, de Figueras GC, Rosselló-Móra R, González-Pastor JE. Salt resistance genes revealed by functional metagenomics from brines and moderate-salinity rhizosphere within a hypersaline environment. Frontiers in Microbiology. 2015;**6**:1-16

[12] Elleuche S, Schäfers C, Blank S, Schröder C, Antranikian G. Exploration of extremophiles for high temperature biotechnological processes. Current Opinion in Microbiology. 2015;**25**:113-119. DOI: 10.1016/j.mib.2015.05.011

[13] Rodrigo-Baños M, Garbayo I, Vílchez C, Bonete MJ, Martínez-Espinosa RM. Carotenoids from haloarchaea and their potential in biotechnology. Marine Drugs. 2015;**13**:5508-5532. DOI: 10.3390/md13095508

[14] Alsafadi D, Al-Mashaqbeh O. A one-stage cultivation process for the production of poly-3-(hydroxybutyrate-co-hydroxyvalerate) from olive mill wastewater by *Haloferax mediterranei*. New Biotechnology. 2017;**34**:47-53

[15] O'Connor EM, Shand RF. Halocins and sulfolobicins: The emerging story of archaeal protein and peptide antibiotics. Journal of Industrial Microbiology and Biotechnology. 2002;**28**:23-31

[16] Delgado-Vargas F, Jiménez AR, Paredes-López O. Natural pigments: Carotenoids, anthocyanins, and betalains—characteristics, biosynthesis, processing, and stability. Critical Reviews in Food Science and Nutrition. 2000;**40**:173-289

[17] Zhang J, Sun Z, Sun P, Chen T, Chen F. Microalgal carotenoids: Beneficial effects and potential in human health. Food and Function. 2014;**5**:413-425

[18] Fiedor J, Burda K. Potential role of carotenoids as antioxidants in human health and disease. Nutrients. 2014;**6**:466-488

[19] Vílchez C, Forján E, Cuaresma M, Bédmar F, Garbayo I, Vega JM. Marine carotenoids: Biological functions and commercial applications. Marine Drugs. 2011;**9**:319-333

[20] Nisar N, Li L, Lu S, Khin NC, Pogson BJ. Carotenoid metabolism in plants. Molecular Plant. 2015;**8**:68-82

[21] Yatsunami R, Ando A, Yang Y, Takaichi S, Kohno M, Matsumura Y, Ikeda H, Fukui T, Nakasone K, Fujita N, Sekine M, Takashina T, Nakamura S. Identification of carotenoids from the extremely halophilic archaeon *Haloarcula japonica*. Frontiers in Microbiology. 2014;**5**:100-105

[22] Mata-Gómez LC, Montañez JC, Méndez-Zavala A, Aguilar CN. Biotechnological production of carotenoids by yeasts: An overview. Microbial Cell Factories. 2014;**13**:1-11

[23] Cunningham FX, Gantt E. Genes and enzymes of carotenoid biosynthesis in plants. Annual Review of Plant Physiology and Plant Molecular Biology. 1998;**49**:557-583

[24] Rao AV, Rao LG. Carotenoids and human health. Pharmacological Research. 2007; **55**:207-216

[25] Del Campo JA, García-González M, Guerrero MG. Outdoor cultivation of microalgae for carotenoid production: Current state and perspectives. Applied Microbiology and Biotechnology. 2007;**74**:1163-1174

[26] Rivera SM, Canela-Garayoa R. Analytical tools for the analysis of carotenoids in diverse materials. Journal of Chromatography A. 2012;**1224**:1-10

[27] Fassett RG, Coombes JS. Astaxanthin in cardiovascular health and disease. Molecules. 2012;**17**:2030-2048

[28] Palczewski G, Amengual J, Hoppel CL, von Lintig J. Evidence for compartmentalization of mammalian carotenoid metabolism. The FASEB Journal. 2014;**28**:4457-4469

[29] Naziri D, Hamidi M, Hassanzadeh S, Vahideh T, Zanjani BM, Nazemyieh H, Hejazi MA, Hejazi MS. Analysis of carotenoid production by *Halorubrum* sp. TBZ126: An extremely halophilic archaeon from Urmia Lake. Advanced Pharmaceutical Bulletin. 2014;**4**:61-67

[30] Kelly M, Jensen SL. Bacterial carotenoids. XXVI. C_{50}-carotenoids. 2. Bacterioruberin. Acta Chemica Scandinavica. 1967;**21**(9):2578-2580

[31] Kushwaha SC, Kramer JK, Kates M. Isolation and characterization of C50-carotenoid pigments and other polar isoprenoids from *Halobacterium cutirubrum*. Biochimica et Biophysica Acta. 1975;**398**:303-314

[32] Jehlicka J, Edwards HG, Oren A. Bacterioruberin and salinixanthin carotenoids of extremely halophilic archaea and bacteria: A Raman spectroscopic study. Spectrochimica Acta Part A: Molecular and Biomolecular Spectroscopy. 2013;**106**:99-103

[33] Bidle KA, Hanson TE, Howell K, Nannen J. HMG-CoA reductase is regulated by salinity at the level of transcription in *Haloferax volcanii*. Extremophiles. 2007;**11**:49-55

[34] Shand RF, Betlach MC. Expression of the bop gene cluster of *Halobacterium halobium* is induced by low oxygen tension and by light. Journal of Bacteriology. 1991;**173**:4692-4699

[35] El-Sayed WS, Takaichi S, Saida H, Kamekura M, Abu-Shady M, Seki H, Kuwabara T. Effects of light and low oxygen tension on pigment biosynthesis in *Halobacterium salinarum*, revealed by a novel method to quantify both retinal and carotenoids. Plant & Cell Physiology. 2002;**43**:379-383

[36] D'Souza SE, Altekar W, D'Souza SF. Adaptive response of *Haloferax mediterranei* to low concentrations of NaCl (<20%) in the growth medium. Archives of Microbiology. 1997;**168**:68-71

[37] Raghavan TM, Furtado I. Expression of carotenoid pigments of haloarchaeal cultures exposed to aniline. Environmental Toxicology. 2005;**20**(2):165-169

[38] Lobasso S, Lopalco P, Mascolo G, Corcelli A. Lipids of the ultra-thin square halophilic archaeon *Haloquadratum walsbyi*. Archaea. 2008;**2**:177-183

[39] Fang CJ, Ku KL, Lee MH, Su NW. Influence of nutritive factors on C_{50} carotenoids production by *Haloferax mediterranei* ATCC 33500 with two-stage cultivation. Bioresource Technology. 2010;**101**:6487-6493

[40] Asker D, Awad T, Ohta Y. Lipids of *Haloferax alexandrinus* strain TMT: An extremely halophilic canthaxanthin-producing archaeon. Journal of Bioscience and Bioengineering. 2002;**93**:37-43

[41] DasSarma S, DasSarma P. Halophiles and their enzymes: Negativity put to good use. Current Opinion in Microbiology. 2015;**25**:120-126

[42] Britton KL, Baker PJ, Fisher M, Ruzheinikov S, Gilmour DJ, Bonete M-J, Ferrer J, Pire C, Esclapez J, Rice DW. Analysis of protein solvent interactions in glucose dehydrogenase from the extreme halophile *Haloferax mediterranei*. Proceedings of the National Academy of Sciences of the United States of America. 2006;**103**:4846-4851

[43] Eichler J. Biotechnological uses of archaeal extremozymes. Biotechnology Advances. 2001;**19**:261-278

[44] Munawar N, Engel PC. Halophilic enzymes: Characteristics, structural adaptation and potential applications for biocatalysis. Current Biotechnology. 2013;**2**:334-344

[45] Hutcheon GW, Vasisht N, Bolhuis A. Characterisation of a highly stable α-amylase from the halophilic archaeon *Haloarcula hispanica*. Extremophiles. 2005;**9**:487-495

[46] Kim J, Dordick JS. Unusual salt and solvent dependence of a protease from an extreme halophile. Biotechnology and Bioengineering. 1997;**55**:471-479

[47] Marhuenda-Egea FC, Bonete MJ. Extreme halophilic enzymes in organic solvents. Current Opinion in Biotechnology. 2002;**13**:385-389

[48] Pire C, Marhuenda-Egea FC, Esclapez J, Alcaraz L, Ferrer J, Bonete MJ. Stability and enzymatic studies of glucose dehydrogenase from the archaeon *Haloferax mediterranei* in reverse micelles. Biocatalysis and Biotransformation. 2004;**22**:17-23

[49] Henrissat B, Bairoch A. New families in the classification of glycosyl hydrolases based on amino acid sequence similarities. Biochemical Journal. 1993;**293**:781-788

[50] Elleuche S, Schröder C, Sahm K, Antranikian G. Extremozymes—biocatalysts with unique properties from extremophilic microorganisms. Current Opinion in Biotechnology. 2014;**29**:116-123

[51] Labes A, Karlsson EN, Fridjonsson OH, Turner P, Hreggvidson GO, Kristjansson JK, Holst O, Schönheit P. Novel members of glycoside hydrolase family 13 derived from environmental DNA. Applied and Environmental Microbiology. 2008;**74**:1914-1921

[52] Good WA, Hartman PA. Properties of the amylase from *Halobacterium halobium*. Journal of Bacteriology. 1970;**104**:601-603

[53] Kobayashi T, Kanai H, Hayashi T, Akiba T, Akaboshi R, Horikoshi K. Haloalkaliphilic maltotriose-forming alpha-amylase from the archaebacterium *Natronococcus* sp. strain Ah-36. Journal of Bacteriology. 1992;**174**:3439-3444

[54] Kobayashi T, Kanai H, Aono R, Horikoshi K, Kudo T. Cloning, expression, and nucleotide sequence of the alpha-amylase gene from the haloalkaliphilic archaeon *Natronococcus* sp. strain Ah-36. Journal of Bacteriology. 1994;**176**(16):5131-5134

[55] Pérez-Pomares F, Bautista V, Ferrer J, Pire C, Marhuenda-Egea FC, Bonete MJ. α-amylase activity from the halophilic archaeon *Haloferax mediterranei*. Extremophiles. 2003;**7**: 299-306

[56] Bautista V, Esclapez J, Pérez-Pomares F, Martínez-Espinosa RM, Camacho M, Bonete MJ. Cyclodextrin glycosyltransferase: A key enzyme in the assimilation of starch by the halophilic archaeon *Haloferax mediterranei*. Extremophiles. 2012;**16**:147-159

[57] Zhang T, Datta S, Eichler J, Ivanova N, Axen SD, Kerfeld CA, Chen F, Kyrpides N, Hugenholtz P, Cheng J-F, Sale KL, Simmons B, Rubin E. Identification of a haloalkaliphilic and thermostable cellulase with improved ionic liquid tolerance. Green Chemistry. 2011;**13**:2083-2090

[58] Li X, Yu HY. Characterization of a halostable endoglucanase with organic solvent-tolerant property from *Haloarcula* sp. G10. International Journal of Biological Macromolecules. 2013;**62**:101-106

[59] Li X, Yu HY. Halostable cellulase with organic solvent tolerance from *Haloarcula* sp. LLSG7 and its application in bioethanol fermentation using agricultural wastes. Journal of Industrial Microbiology and Biotechnology. 2013;**40**:1357-1365

[60] Sorokin DY, Toshchakov SV, Kolganova TV, Kublanov IV. Halo(natrono)archaea isolated from hypersaline lakes utilize cellulose and chitin as growth substrates. Frontiers in Microbiology. 2015;**6**:942

[61] Dahiya N, Tewari R, Hoondal GS. Biotechnological aspects of chitinolytic enzymes: A review. Applied Microbiology and Biotechnology. 2006;**71**:773-782

[62] Hou J, Han J, Cai L, Zhou J, Lü Y, Jin C, Liu J, Xiang H. Characterization of genes for chitin catabolism in *Haloferax mediterranei*. Applied Microbiology and Biotechnology. 2014;**98**:1185-1194

[63] Adrio J, Demain A. Microbial enzymes: Tools for biotechnological processes. Biomolecules. 2014;**4**:117-139

[64] Białkowska A, Gromek E, Florczak T, Krysiak J, Szulczewska K, Turkiewicz M. Extremophilic proteases: Developments of their special functions, potential resources and biotechnological applications. In: Rampelotto PH, editor. Biotechnology of Extremophiles. Springer International Publishing; Switzerland. 2016. pp. 399-444

[65] Capiralla H, Hiroi T, Hirokawa T, Maeda S. Purification and characterization of a hydrophobic amino acid—specific endopeptidase from *Halobacterium halobium* S9 with potential application in debittering of protein hydrolysates. Process Biochemistry. 2002;**38**:571-579

[66] Schmitt W, Rdest U, Goebel W. Efficient high-performance liquid chromatographic system for the purification of a halobacterial serine protease. Journal of Chromatography A. 1990;**521**(2):211-220

[67] Marhuenda-Egea FC, Piera-Velázquez S, Cadenas C, Cadenas E. An extreme halophilic enzyme active at low salt in reversed micelles. Journal of Biotechnology. 2002;**93**:159-164

[68] Anobom CD, Pinheiro AS, De-Andrade RA, Aguieiras ECG, Andrade GC, Moura MV, Almeida RV, Freire DM. From structure to catalysis: Recent developments in the biotechnological applications of lipases. Biomed Research International. 2014;**2014**:1-11

[69] Schreck SD, Grunden AM. Biotechnological applications of halophilic lipases and thioesterases. Applied Microbiology and Biotechnology. 2014;**98**:1011-1021

[70] Bhatnagar T, Boutaiba S, Hacene H, Cayol J-L, Fardeau M-L, Ollivier B, Baratti JC. Lipolytic activity from Halobacteria: Screening and hydrolase production. FEMS Microbiology Letters. 2006;248(2):133-140

[71] Boutaiba S, Bhatnagar T, Hacene H, Mitchell DA, Baratti JC. Preliminary characterisation of a lipolytic activity from an extremely halophilic archaeon, *Natronococcus* sp. Journal of Molecular Catalysis B: Enzymatic. 2006;**41**(1-2):21-26

[72] Ozcan B, Ozyilmaz G, Cokmus C, Caliskan M. Characterization of extracellular esterase and lipase activities from five halophilic archaeal strains. Journal of Industrial Microbiology and Biotechnology. 2009;**36**(1):105-110

[73] Camacho RM, Mateos JC, González-Reynoso O, Prado LA, Córdova J. Production and characterization of esterase and lipase from *Haloarcula marismortui*. Journal of Industrial Microbiology and Biotechnology. 2009;**36**(7):901-909

[74] Müller-Santos M, de Souza EM, Pedrosa FDO, Mitchell DA, Longhi S, Carrière F, Canaan S, Krieger N. First evidence for the salt-dependent folding and activity of an esterase from the halophilic archaea *Haloarcula marismortui*. Biochimica et Biophysica Acta (BBA)-Molecular and Cell Biology of Lipids. 2009;**1791**(8):719-729

[75] Li X, Yu HY. Characterization of an organic solvent-tolerant lipase from *Haloarcula* sp. G41 and its application for biodiesel production. Folia Microbiologica. 2014;**59**(6):455-463

[76] Poli A, Di Donato P, Abbamondi GR, Nicolaus B. Synthesis, production, and biotechnological applications of exopolysaccharides and polyhydroxyalkanoates by archaea. Archaea. 2011;**2011**:693253. DOI: 10.1155/2011/693253

[77] Mozejko-Ciesielska J, Kiewisz R. Bacterial polyhydroxyalkanoates: Still fabulous? Microbial Research. 2016;**192**:271-282

[78] Meng DC, Shen R, Yao H, Chen JC, Wu Q, Chen GQ. Engineering the diversity of polyesters. Current Opinion in Biotechnology. 2014;**29**:24-33

[79] Olivera ER, Arcos M, Naharro G, Luengo JM. Unusual PHA biosynthesis. In: Chen GQ, editor. Plastics from Bacteria: Natural Functions and Applications, Microbiology Monographs. 1st ed. Springer; Berlin Heidelberg. 2010. pp. 133-186

[80] Rehm BH. Polyester synthases: Natural catalysts for plastics. Biochemical Journal. 2003; **376**:15-33

[81] McCool GJ, Cannon MC. PhaC and PhaR are required for polyhydroxyalkanoic acid synthase activity in *Bacillus megaterium*. Journal of Bacteriology. 2001;**183**(14):4235-4243

[82] Han J, Lu Q, Zhou L, Zhou J, Xiang H. Molecular characterization of the phaECHm genes, required for biosynthesis of poly(3-hydroxybutyrate) in the extremely halophilic archaeon *Haloarcula marismortui*. Applied and Environmental Microbiology. 2007;**73**(19):6058-6065

[83] Lu Q, Han J, Zhou L, Zhou J, Xiang H. Genetic and biochemical characterization of the poly(3-hydroxybutyrate-co-3-hydroxyvalerate) synthase in *Haloferax mediterranei*. Journal of Bacteriology. 2008;**190**(12):4173-4180

[84] Don TM, Chen CW, Chan TH. Preparation and characterization of poly(hydroxyalkanoate) from the fermentation of *Haloferax mediterranei*. Journal of Biomaterials Science, Polymer Edition. 2006;**17**(12):1425-1438

[85] Taran M, Amirkhani H. Strategies of poly(3-hydroxybutyrate) synthesis by *Haloarcula* sp. IRU1 utilizing glucose as a carbon source: Optimization of culture conditions by Taguchi methodology. International Journal of Biological Macromolecules. 2010;**47**:632-634

[86] Fernández-Castillo R, Rodríguez-Valera F, González-Ramos J, Ruiz-Berraquero F. Accumulation of poly(β-hydroxybutyrate) by halobacteria. Applied and Environmental Microbiology. 1986;**51**(1):214-216

[87] Koller M, Hesse P, Bona R, Kutschera C, Atlic A, Braunegg G. Potential of various archaea and eubacterial strains as industrial polyhydroxyalkanoate producers from whey. Macromolecular Bioscience. 2007;**7**:218-226

[88] Koller M, Hesse P, Bona R, Kutschera C, Atlic A, Braunegg G. Biosynthesis of high quality polyhydroxyalkanoate co- and terpolyesters for potential medical application by the archaeon *Haloferax mediterranei*. Macromolecular Symposia. 2007;**253**:33-39

[89] Cavalheiro JM, Raposo RS, de Almeida MC, Cesário MT, Sevrin C, Grandfils C, da Fonseca MM. Effect of cultivation parameters on the production of poly(3-hydroxybutyrate-co-4-hydroxybutyrate) and poly(3-hydroxybutyrate-4-hydroxybutyrate-3-hydroxyvalerate) by *Cupriavidus necator* using waste glycerol. Bioresource Technology. 2012;**111**:391-397

[90] Hermann-Krauss C, Koller M, Muhr A, Fasl H, Stelzer F, Braunegg G. Archaeal production of polyhydroxyalkanoate (PHA) co- and terpolyesters from biodiesel industry-derived by-products. Archaea. 2013;**2013**:129268. DOI: 10.1155/2013/129268

[91] Huang TY, Duan KJ, Huang SY, Chen CW. Production of polyhydroxyalkanoates from inexpensive extruded rice bran and starch by *Haloferax mediterranei*. Journal of Industrial Microbiology and Biotechnology. 2006;**33**:701-706

[92] Bhattacharyya A, Saha J, Haldar S, Bhowmic A, Mukhopadhyay UK, Mukherjee J. Production of poly-3-(hydroxybutyrate-co-hydroxyvalerate) by *Haloferax mediterranei* using rice-based ethanol stillage with simultaneous recovery and re-use of medium salts. Extremophiles. 2014;**18**:463-470

[93] Pais J, Serafim LS, Freitas F, Reis MAM. Conversion of cheese whey into poly(3-hydroxybutyrate-co-3-hydroxyvalerate) by *Haloferax mediterranei*. New Biotechnology. 2016;**33** (1):224-230

[94] Dionisi D, Carucci G, Papini MP, Riccardi C, Majone M, Carrasco F. Olive oil mil effluents as a feedstock for production of biodegradable polymers. Water Research. 2005;**39**:2076-2084

[95] Beccari M, Bertin L, Dionisi D, Fava F, Lampis S, Majone M, Valentino F, Vallini G, Villano M. Exploiting olive oil mill effluents as a renewable resource for production of biodegradable polymers through a combined anaerobic-aerobic process. Journal of Chemical Technology and Biotechnology. 2009;**84**:901-908

[96] Choi HJ, Kim J, Jhon MS. Viscoelastic characterization of biodegradable poly(3-hydroxybutyrate-co-3-hydroxyvalerate). Polymer. 1999;**40**(14):4135-4138

[97] Quillaguamán J, Guzmán H, Van-Thuoc D, Hatti-Kaul R. Synthesis and production of polyhydroxyalkanoates by halophiles: Current potential and future prospects. Applied Microbiology and Biotechnology. 2010;**85**:1687-1696

[98] Bugnicourt E, Cinelli P, Lazzeri A, Álvarez V. Polyhydroxyalkanoate (PHA): Review of synthesis, characteristics, processing and potential applications in packaging. Express Polymer Letters. 2014;**8**(11):791-808

[99] Wang Y, Yin J, Chen GQ. Polyhydroxyalkanoates, challenges and opportunities. Current Opinion in Biotechnology. 2014;**30**:59-65

[100] Laycock B, Halley P, Pratt S, Werker A, Lant P. The petrochemical properties of microbial polyhydroxyalkanoates. Progress in Polymer Science. 2013;**38**:536-583

[101] Meseguer I, Torreblanca M, Konishi T. Specific inhibition of the halobacterial Na^+/H^+ antiporter by halocin H6. Journal of Biological Chemistry. 1995;**270**:6450-6455

[102] Besse A, Peduzzi J, Rebuffat S, Carré-Mlouka A. Antimicrobial peptides and proteins in the face of extremes: Lessons from archaeocins. Biochimie. 2015;**118**:344-355. DOI: 10.1016/j.biochi.2015.06.004

[103] Nájera-Fernández C, Zafrilla B, Bonete MJ, Martínez-Espinosa RM. Role of the denitrifying haloarchaea in the treatment of nitrite-brines. International Microbiology. 2012;**15**:111-119

Chapter 5

Plasmid Curing is a Promising Approach to Improve Thermophiles for Biotechnological Applications: Perspectives in *Archaea*

Tatsuki Mizuno, Takashi Ohshiro and
Hirokazu Suzuki

Additional information is available at the end of the chapter

http://dx.doi.org/10.5772/intechopen.70041

Abstract

Thermophiles are attractive as host cells for microbial processes to produce or degrade various compounds. In these applications, it is often desirable to improve the properties of thermophiles, such as their growth rate, cell density, and protein productivity, although this is rarely achieved because of the lack of general approaches. In this chapter, we describe the elimination of the pHTA426 plasmid from a moderate thermophile, *Geobacillus kaustophilus* HTA426, and its effects on the microbial properties. This process, called plasmid curing, was simply achieved using a DNA intercalator and confirmed by phenotypic and genotypic analyses. Of note, pHTA426 curing had beneficial effects on diverse properties, probably because of the reduced energy burden in terms of plasmid replication at high temperatures. The result suggests that plasmid curing is a simple and versatile approach for improving thermophiles. In particular, this approach may be effective for archaeal thermophiles because they grow at much higher temperatures and could have the greater energy burden on plasmid replication. Data mining has also shown that plasmids are distributed in archaeal thermophiles. This chapter provides a new tip for improving archaeal thermophiles, thereby increasing the opportunities for their use in various biotechnological applications.

Keywords: genetic engineering, host improvement, plasmid curing, plasmid elimination, thermophile application

1. Introduction

Thermophiles are organisms that are capable of growing at temperatures above 55°C. Archaeal thermophiles generally grow at much higher temperatures and thus comprise most extreme thermophiles and hyperthermophiles. These thermophiles are attractive organisms in biotechnological applications because they produce thermostable enzymes, which can be used as stable industrial catalysts even at high temperatures. Thermophile cells themselves are attractive as hosts for microbial processes at high temperatures.

High-temperature processes have several advantages compared with moderate processes using mesophiles, where an important advantage is that high temperature prevents the growth of animal pathogens, including all viruses, which are killed or at least prevented from proliferating at temperatures above 65°C [1]. High temperature also inhibits growth and/or metabolism by mesophiles, which may hinder processes of interests via involuntary reactions. The advantage is especially important for processes using crude biomass (e.g., sewage, municipal or agricultural waste, and materials from animal farms) because mesophiles and virulent pathogens are common in biomass from natural environments and they may increase during reactions performed under moderate conditions. In addition, high temperature facilitates the removal of volatile products (e.g., ethanol and butanol) while decreasing oxygen solubility; therefore, thermophiles are practical for fermentative production of alcohols [2–6]. Moreover, thermophiles often have remarkable properties useful for bioprocesses. A good example is the hyperthermophilic archaeon *Thermococcus kodakarensis* KOD1, which can use protons as an electron accepter in catabolism to generate molecular hydrogen and has been studied as a hydrogen production tool [7].

In this chapter, we will demonstrate the salutary effects of plasmid curing on thermophiles using as an example a prokaryotic thermophile that was isolated from deep sea sediments of the Mariana Trench, *Geobacillus kaustophilus* HTA426 [8, 9]. Its growth occurs at temperatures

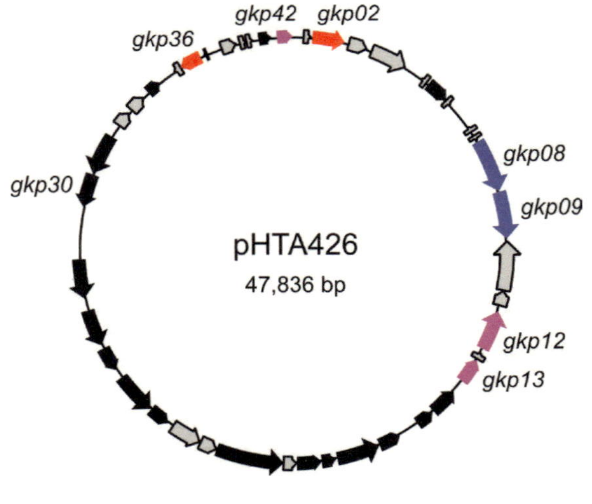

Figure 1. Structure of pHTA426. Genes for possible and hypothetical proteins are indicated by solid and faded arrows, respectively. The plasmid contains possible genes responsible for plasmid replication (*gkp02 and gkp36*), DNA restriction–modification (*gkp08 and gkp09*), and integrase/transposase (*gkp12 and gkp13*).

ranging between 42 and 74°C, with optimal growth at 60°C, and is as rapid as *Escherichia coli* and *Bacillus subtilis*. Genetic tools are available for this strain [10–16]. The whole genome sequence has been determined [17], showing that *G. kaustophilus* HTA426 harbors the circular plasmid pHTA426 (**Figure 1**). Because the members of the genus *Geobacillus* include strains that are useful for high-temperature processes, as demonstrated by strains that are capable of degrading hydrocarbons [18], long-chain alkanes [19–21], biphenyls [22], paraffin-wax [23], or nylons [24], we have studied biotechnological applications of the genus using *G. kaustophilus* HTA426 as a model and pilot strain.

Aiming to construct a plasmid-free strain that may be useful for the genetic analysis of pHTA426, this study was originally designed to eliminate this plasmid from an HTA426 derivative, *G. kaustophilus* MK244. The resultant strain MK633 was then characterized to confirm that plasmid elimination (termed plasmid curing) had no effects on its microbial properties, but the analysis unexpectedly demonstrated that *G. kaustophilus* MK633 had advantages compared with the parent strain MK244 in terms of several properties. We suggest here that plasmid curing is a promising approach for improving diverse thermophiles.

2. Experimental procedures

2.1. Bacterial strains and culture conditions

The bacterial strains employed are summarized in **Table 1**. *G. kaustophilus* MK244 was previously constructed from *G. kaustophilus* HTA426 [14]. If not specified otherwise, *G. kaustophilus* strains were grown at 60°C in Luria–Bertani (LB) and minimal media (MM) with rotary shaking at 180 rpm. MM comprised 0.3 g l^{-1} K_2SO_4, 2.5 g l^{-1} $Na_2HPO_4 \cdot 12H_2O$, 1 g l^{-1} NH_4Cl, 0.4 g l^{-1} $MgSO_4$, 3 mg l^{-1} $MnCl_2 \cdot 4H_2O$, 5 mg l^{-1} $CaCl_2 \cdot 2H_2O$, 7 mg l^{-1} $FeCl_3 \cdot 6H_2O$, 0.1% trace element solution [25], 10 mM Tris-HCl (pH 7.0), 1 g l^{-1} casamino acids, and 10 g l^{-1} D-glucose. The media also contained 5 mg l^{-1} kanamycin, 10 mg l^{-1} uracil, 50 mg l^{-1} 5-fluoroorotic acid, 1 g l^{-1} yeast extract, and/or 50 mg l^{-1} 5-bromo-4-chloro-3-indolyl-β-D-galactopyranoside (X-gal), as necessary. *E. coli* strains were grown at 37°C in LB medium supplemented with appropriate antibiotics (50 mg l^{-1} ampicillin, 50 mg l^{-1} kanamycin, 13 mg l^{-1} chloramphenicol, and/or 7 mg l^{-1} tetracycline). The optical cell density at 600 nm was monitored automatically using an OD-MonitorA instrument (Taitec, Saitama, Japan).

2.2. Plasmids

The *E. coli-Geobacillus* shuttle plasmids are summarized in **Table 2**. To construct the pGKE25-*bgaB* plasmid, a *gkp09* downstream region of pHTA426 was amplified using the primers 5′-GGAGTTTGCCAAACTCCGGATCCAGCTTGGATTTATC-3′ (*Bam*HI site underlined) and 5′-CACAAGCTTGGGGCTGGATGTAATG-3′ (*Hin*dIII site underlined), and a *gkp09* upstream region was amplified using the primers 5′-GGCGGATCCTTCCGATTAGGTTCCCATGC-3′ (*Bam*HI site underlined) and 5′-GGCGAATTCGGCCTTTTCGCATTAC-3′ (*Eco*RI site

Strain	Relevant description	Reference
E. coli		
BR397	Conjugation helper strain; F^- e14$^-$ (*mcrA*$^-$) Δ(*mrr-hsdRMS-mcrBC*)114::*IS10* Δ*dcm*::*lacZ* Δ*dam*::*metB* pUB307 pIR207	[18]
BR398	Conjugation helper strain; F^- e14$^-$ (*mcrA*$^-$) Δ(*mrr-hsdRMS-mcrBC*)114::*IS10* Δ*dcm*::*lacZ* pUB307 pIR207	[18]
BR408	Conjugation helper strain; F^- e14$^-$ (*mcrA*$^-$) Δ(*mrr-hsdRMS-mcrBC*)114::*IS10* Δ*dcm*::*lacZ* pUB307 pIR408	[18]
G. kaustophilus		
MK244	Derivative of the wild-type strain HTA426; Δ*pyrF* Δ*pyrR* Δ$hsdM_1S_1R_1$ Δ($mcrB_1$-$mcrB_2$-$hsdM_2S_2R_2$-*mrr*) pHTA426	[20]
MK244′	Derivative of the MK244 strain; Δ*pyrF* Δ*pyrR* Δ$hsdM_1S_1R_1$ Δ($mcrB_1$-$mcrB_2$-$hsdM_2S_2R_2$-*mrr*) pHTA426 (Δ*gkp09*::P_{sigA}-*bgaB*)	This study
$MK244_{bgaB}$	Derivative of the MK244 strain; Δ*pyrF* Δ*pyrR* Δ$hsdM_1S_1R_1$ Δ($mcrB_1$-$mcrB_2$-$hsdM_2S_2R_2$-*mrr*) *gk0707*::P_{gk704}-*bgaB* pHTA426	This study
MK633	Derivative of the MK244 strain; Δ*pyrF* Δ*pyrR* Δ$hsdM_1S_1R_1$ Δ($mcrB_1$-$mcrB_2$-$hsdM_2S_2R_2$-*mrr*)	This study
$MK633_{bgaB}$	Derivative of the MK633 strain; Δ*pyrF* Δ*pyrR* Δ$hsdM_1S_1R_1$ Δ($mcrB_1$-$mcrB_2$-$hsdM_2S_2R_2$-*mrr*) *gk0707*::P_{gk704}-*bgaB*	This study

Table 1. Bacterial strains used in this study. pUB307 mediates the conjugative transfer of *oriT*-containing plasmids. This plasmid contains kanamycin and tetracycline resistance genes. pIR207 is a chloramphenicol resistance plasmid derived from pACYCDuet-1 (Merck KgaA, Darmstadt, Germany). The plasmid was used to construct pIR408, which contains the $hsdM_1S_1$ and $hsdM_2S_2$ genes from *G. kaustophilus* HTA426, and thus, it is responsible for heterologous DNA methylation in *E. coli* [18]. *G. kaustophilus* MK244 lacks genes related to pyrimidine biosynthesis (*pyrF* and *pyrR*) and DNA restriction–modification ($hsdM_1S_1R_1$, $mcrB_1$, $mcrB_2$, $hsdM_2S_2R_2$, and *mrr*). P_{sigA}-*bgaB* and P_{gk704}-*bgaB* denote *bgaB* expression cassettes under the control of P_{sigA} [19] and P_{gk704} promoters [21], respectively.

Plasmid	Relevant description	Reference
pGAM47-*bgaB*	pUC19 derivative; pUC replicon, *oriT, bla, pyrF*, P_{sigA}-*bgaB* flanked by *gk0707* upstream and downstream regions	[19]
pGAM48-*bgaB*	pUC19 derivative; pUC replicon, *oriT, bla, pyrF*, P_{gk704}-*bgaB* flanked by *gk0707* upstream and downstream regions	[21]
pGKE25	pUC19 derivative; pUC replicon, *oriT, bla, pyrF*	[20]
pGKE25-*bgaB*	pGKE25 derivative; pUC replicon, *oriT, bla, pyrF*, P_{sigA}-*bgaB* flanked by *gkp09* upstream and downstream regions	This study
pUCG18T	pUC18 derivative; pUC and pBST1 replicons, *oriT, bla, TK101*	[18]

Table 2. *E. coli-Geobacillus* shuttle plasmids used in this study. *bla* and *TK101* genes confer resistance to ampicillin in *E. coli* and kanamycin in *G. kaustophilus*, respectively. *pyrF* encodes orotidine-5′-phosphate decarboxylase in *G. kaustophilus* HTA426. *oriT* is the conjugative transfer origin. P_{sigA}-*bgaB* and P_{gk704}-*bgaB* denote *bgaB* expression cassettes under the control of P_{sigA} [19] and P_{gk704} promoters [21], respectively. The pUC and pBST1 replicons allow autonomous plasmid replication in *E. coli* and *G. kaustophilus*, respectively.

underlined). In addition, a *bgaB* expression cassette encoding thermostable β-galactosidase under the control of P_{sigA} promoter was amplified from the pGAM47-*bgaB* plasmid [13] using the primers 5′-AAGATCTCTTCGCCTCATCCGCACGATTTC-3′ and 5′-GCCAGATCTCTAAACCTTCCCGGCTTCATC-3′ (*Bgl*II site underlined). The downstream region was cloned between the *Bam*HI and *Hind*III sites of the pGKE25 plasmid [14], and the upstream region was cloned between the *Bam*HI and *Eco*RI sites. The *bgaB* expression cassette was then cloned in the *Bam*HI site of the resulting plasmid to yield pGKE25-*bgaB* for replacing the *gkp09* gene in pHTA426 with the *bgaB* cassette. The pGAM48-*bgaB* plasmid [15] was used to integrate a *bgaB* expression cassette under the control of the P_{gk704} promoter at the *gk0707* locus in the *G. kaustophilus* chromosome. The pUCG18T plasmid [12] was used to assess the transformation efficiency of *G. kaustophilus*.

2.3. Plasmid introduction into *G. kaustophilus*

Plasmids were introduced into *G. kaustophilus* by conjugative plasmid transfer from *E. coli* BR408 [12]. Briefly, an *E. coli* donor (10 ml) and a *G. kaustophilus* recipient (100 ml) were grown in LB media. The cells were subsequently mixed, centrifuged, and spotted onto LB plates. After incubation at 37°C for 20 h, the resultant cells were collected and incubated at 60°C on appropriate media to isolate *G. kaustophilus* transformants. The transformation efficiency, as the number of transformants per 10^6 recipients, was determined as described previously [12]. Data were expressed as the mean ± standard error ($n = 3$).

2.4. pHTA426 curing from *G. kaustophilus* MK244

The *gkp09* gene in pHTA426 was replaced by a *bgaB* expression cassette using pGKE25-*bgaB* with *pyrF*-based counterselection [13]. The resultant clone, strain MK244′, was successively cultured three times in LB media supplemented with 20 μM acridine orange to facilitate pHTA426 curing. In each culture, an aliquot (10^3 cells) was grown on LB plates supplemented with X-gal to identify candidates from which pHTA426 was eliminated along with the *bgaB* cassette. The candidates were purified using LB plates with X-gal.

2.5. Southern blot

Total DNA (25 μg) was digested using *Eco*RV and separated on an agarose gel by electrophoresis. DNA was transferred onto a nylon membrane and hybridized with digoxigenin-labeled DNA probes to detect the *bgaB* and *gkp30* regions. Probes were synthesized using PCR DIG Probe Synthesis Kit (Roche, Basel, Switzerland) using the primers 5′-GCCGGATCCTGTTATCCTCAATTTGTTAC-3′ and 5′-GCCGGATCCTGTTATCCTCAATTTGTTAC-3′ (for *bgaB* probe) and 5′-CCGATATAGGCTGAGAACGC-3′ and 5′-CAGCTGGTAGACATGGGG-3′ (for *gkp30* probe). Hybridized DNA was detected with the chromogenic method using DIG Nucleic Acid Detection Kit (Roche).

2.6. Construction of *G. kaustophilus* $MK244_{bgaB}$ and $MK633_{bgaB}$

A *bgaB* expression cassette under the control of the P_{gk704} promoter was integrated at the *gk0707* locus in *G. kaustophilus* using pGAM48-*bgaB*, as described previously [15]. *G. kaustophilus*

MK244 and MK633 were subjected to this process to generate strains MK244$_{bgaB}$ and MK633$_{bgaB}$, respectively.

2.7. BgaB assay

G. kaustophilus MK244$_{bgaB}$ and MK633$_{bgaB}$ were cultured for 4 h in MM containing yeast extract but not D-glucose or casamino acids, and then for 20 h in the presence of 10 g l^{-1} maltose. Cells were subsequently harvested, sonicated in 50 mM sodium phosphate (pH 6.0), and clarified by centrifugation to obtain a lysate. The reaction mixture (100 μl) contained 50 mM sodium phosphate (pH 6.0), 2 mM *p*-nitrophenyl-β-D-galactopyranoside, and the lysate. The mixture was incubated at 60°C to react and then diluted with ice-cold 2 M sodium carbonate (900 μl) to terminate the reaction. *p*-Nitrophenol liberated in the mixture was quantified based on the absorbance at 405 nm and using an experimentally derived standard curve. One unit was defined as the amount of enzyme required to generate 1 μmol of *p*-nitrophenol per min. Proteins were quantified by the Bradford method using a protein assay kit (Nacalai Tesque, Kyoto, Japan). Data were expressed as the mean ± standard error (n = 4–5).

2.8. Plasmid stability assay

G. kaustophilus harboring pUCG18T was precultured in LB medium with kanamycin until the optical cell density at 600 nm reached 0.5. An aliquot (200 μl) was then cultured in LB medium (20 ml) without kanamycin until the stationary phase. The resultant cells were incubated on LB plates with or without kanamycin to determine the concentrations of kanamycin-resistant and viable cells, respectively. The plasmid retention rate was defined as the number of kanamycin-resistant cells per viable cells. Data were expressed as the mean ± standard error (n = 3).

2.9. Cell density assay

G. kaustophilus cells were cultured in LB medium until the stationary phase. Cells were harvested by centrifugation and analyzed to determine the wet weight. Data were expressed as the mean ± standard error (n = 4–5).

2.10. Mutation frequency assay

The frequency of spontaneous mutations was assessed based on the generation of rifampicin- and streptomycin-resistant cells via *rpoB* and *rpsL* genes, respectively [26]. *G. kaustophilus* (10^3 cells) was cultured at 60°C in LB medium until the stationary phase. The resultant cells were then incubated on LB plates with or without efficacious rifampicin or streptomycin (10 mg l^{-1}) to determine the concentrations of mutant (rifampicin- or streptomycin-resistant) and viable cells, respectively. The colonies were counted to calculate the ratio of mutant cells relative to the viable cells incubated, which was defined as the mutation frequency. Data were expressed as the mean ± standard error (n = 3).

2.11. Nucleotide stability assay

Deoxyribonucleoside triphosphates (1 mM) were incubated for 24 h in 20 mM sodium phosphate (pH 7.0) at 30, 60, 80, and 90°C. The residual nucleotides in samples (5 μl) were analyzed using reversed-phase high-performance liquid chromatography. The chromatography system comprised solvent delivery units (LC-10AT; Shimadzu, Kyoto, Japan), an ultraviolet absorption detector (SPD-10Avp; Shimadzu), a reverse-phase column (Cosmosil 2.5C_{18}-MS-II; Nacalai Tesque), and a column bath at 30°C. Solvents A and B comprised 5 mM tetrabutylammonium bromide in 20 mM sodium phosphate (pH 7.0) and 90% (v/v) acetonitrile in water, respectively. After injecting the sample into a column that had been equilibrated with 15% solvent B, the column was isocratically developed at a flow rate of 0.5 ml min^{-1} for 1 min and then at a linear gradient of 15–60% solvent B over 15 min. The chromatogram was obtained by detection at 260 nm.

2.12. Genome data mining

Genome data were collected from the GenBank database (https://www.ncbi.nlm.nih.gov/genome) in December 2016. The collection was performed for bacterial thermophiles (*Geobacillus* spp.), bacterial mesophiles (*B. subtilis*), archaeal thermophiles (*Pyrobaculum, Pyrococcus, Sulfolobus,* and *Thermococcus* spp.), archaeal mesophiles (*Haloarcula, Halococcus, Haloferax,* and *Halorubrum* spp.), and archaeal methanogens (*Methanobacterium, Methanobrevibacter, Methanocaldococcus, Methanocella, Methanococcoides, Methanococcus, Methanocorpusculum, Methanoculleus, Methanofollis, Methanogenium, Methanohalophilus, Methanolacinia, Methanolinea, Methanolobus, Methanomassiliicoccus, Methanomethylovorans, Methanomicrobium, Methanoplanus, Methanoregula, Methanosaeta, Methanosalsum, Methanosarcina, Methanosphaerula, Methanothermobacter, Methanothermococcus, Methanothermus, Methanotorris,* and *Methermicoccus* spp.). The growth temperatures of archaeal methanogens were based on the Methanogens database (http://metanogen.biotech.uni.wroc.pl). Genome sizes were expressed as the mean ± standard deviation.

3. Results

3.1. Genetic features of the pHTA426 plasmid

The pHTA426 sequence suggested that the plasmid was a large circular plasmid (47.9 kb) comprising 1.3% of the circular chromosome of *G. kaustophilus* HTA426 (3.54 Mb) and that it encoded possible proteins for plasmid replication (*gkp02*) and plasmid partition (*gkp36*). A partition system has a role in the stable transmission of single-copy plasmids during cell division, so pHTA426 appeared to be present as a single copy in *G. kaustophilus* HTA426. In addition, the plasmid contained genes for a type II restriction–modification system, which was homologous to the *Alw*I restriction-modification system (*gkp08* encoding methyltransferase and *gkp09* encoding endonuclease). A type II restriction-modification system generally comprises an endonuclease and methyltransferase, where the endonuclease cuts exogenous DNA at specific sites, but not endogenous DNA that has been methylated by methyltransferase. In the *Alw*I system, *Alw*I methyltransferase is responsible for 5′-GG^{6m}ATC-3′ and 5′-G^{6m}ATCC-3′ methylation (^{6m}A, N^6-methyladenin), whereas *Alw*I endonuclease cuts 5′-GGATC-3′ and 5′-GATCC-3′ sites but not 5′-GG^{6m}ATC-3′ and 5′-G^{6m}ATCC-3′ sites. Because plasmids carrying a type II restriction-modification system have greater segregational stability [27], it is likely that the *gkp08–gkp09* system contributes to the stable maintenance of pHTA426.

3.2. Construction of *G. kaustophilus* MK633

Figure 2A shows the process employed to eliminate pHTA426 from *G. kaustophilus* MK244. To facilitate plasmid curing and readily identify positive clones from which pHTA426 was eliminated, the *gkp09* gene was preliminarily replaced by a *bgaB* expression cassette using pGKE25-*bgaB*. The resultant strain MK244′ was then cultured successively in the presence of a DNA intercalator, and we screened for positive clones by using the X-gal degradation assay. Fortunately, one positive clone was obtained from the first culture but not from the second culture. From the third culture, 24 positive clones were identified, which suggests that three successive rounds of culture were effective for pHTA426 curing. The positive clone obtained from the first culture was designated as *G. kaustophilus* MK633.

G. kaustophilus MK244′ degraded X-gal to form blue colonies on LB plates with X-gal, whereas strains MK244 and MK633 did not (**Figure 2B**). This suggests that strain MK633 lacked the *bgaB* gene. The MK633 chromosome is resistant to *Dpn*I (which digests 5′-G^{6m}ATC-3′ but not 5′-GATC-3′) but sensitive to *Alw*I (see above), in contrast to the chromosomes from strains MK244 and MK244′ (**Figure 2C**), so it is likely that strain MK633 lacked the *gkp08* gene encoding an *Alw*I methyltransferase homolog. Southern blot analysis (**Figure 2D**) confirmed that strain MK633 lacked

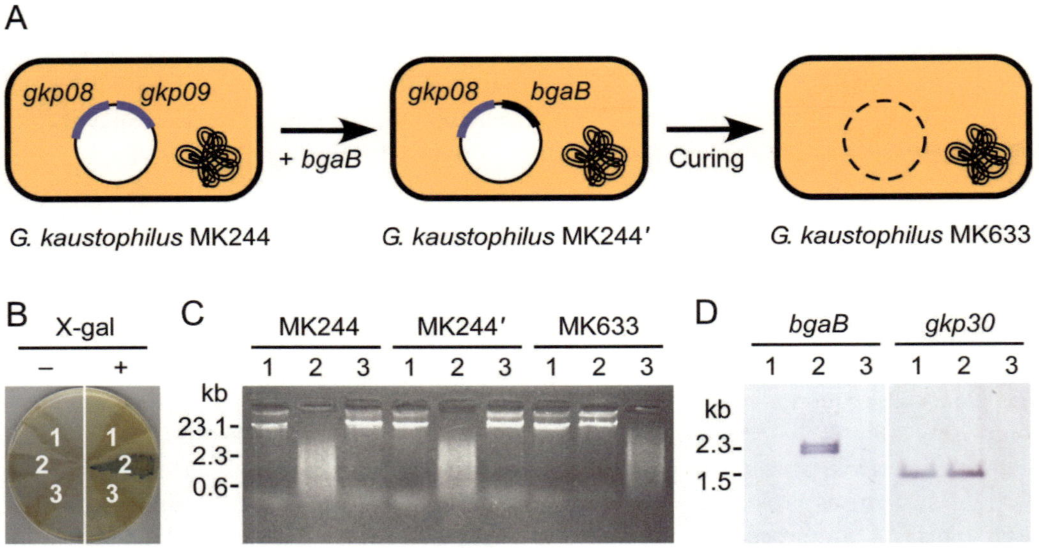

Figure 2. Construction of *G. kaustophilus* MK633. (A) Schematic representation of pHTA426 curing from *G. kaustophilus* MK244. The *gkp09* gene in pHTA426 was replicated by the *bgaB* expression cassette (P_{sigA}-*bgaB*) to generate strain MK244′. The plasmid pHTA426 (Δ*gkp09*::P_{sigA}-*bgaB*) in strain MK244′ was subsequently eliminated using acridine orange. The positive clones from which pHTA426 was eliminated, including strain MK633, were identified using the X-gal degradation assay. (B) X-gal degradation assay. *G. kaustophilus* strains MK244 (1), MK244′ (2), and MK633 (3) were grown at 60°C on LB plates with (+) or without (–) X-gal. (C) DNA methylation assay of MK244, MK244′, and MK633 chromosomes. Total DNA from the strains was digested with restriction enzymes (1, none; 2, *Dpn*I; 3, *Alw*I) and analyzed by agarose gel electrophoresis. (D) Southern blot analysis of pHTA426. Total DNA from strains MK244 (1), MK244′ (2), and MK633 (3) was digested with *Eco*RV, and detected by *bgaB* (left panel) and *gkp30* probes (right panel).

the *bgaB* and *gkp30* genes, which are located on opposite sides of pHTA426 (Δ*gkp09*::P_{sigA}-*bgaB*). Based on these results, we concluded that *G. kaustophilus* MK633 lacked pHTA426.

3.3. Microbial properties of *G. kaustophilus* MK244 and MK633

G. kaustophilus MK244 and MK633 were characterized in detail (**Table 3**). Both strains grew in LB and MM with comparable doubling times. The difference in their mutation frequencies was also not significant. However, strain MK633 was more transformed efficiently with pUCG18T than strain MK244 and it maintained the plasmid with higher stability. Moreover, strain MK633 grew at higher cell densities than strain MK244. The cell density of *G. kaustophilus* MK244′ was lower than that of strain MK633 at 60°C (0.30 ± 0.03 g wet), but the pUCG18T retention rate was comparable (43 ± 14%).

When cultured at 60°C, strain $MK633_{bgaB}$ produced 220 ± 20 units of BgaB, whereas strain $MK244_{bgaB}$ produced 140 ± 10 units (**Figure 3A**). BgaB was also produced more abundantly by $MK633_{bgaB}$ at 50 and 70°C. Moreover, *G. kaustophilus* $MK633_{bgaB}$ had advantages in terms of the cell yield per culture (**Figure 3B**), protein yield per culture (**Figure 3C**), and BgaB-specific activity (**Figure 3D**). The higher specific activity suggests that $MK633_{bgaB}$ enhanced the BgaB productivity per cell.

3.4. Nucleotide stability

In bacteria and *Archaea*, DNA replication proceeds in cytosol (approximately at pH 7) using deoxyribonucleoside triphosphates as the building blocks. To assess their thermolability in cytosol, deoxyribonucleoside triphosphates (i.e., dATP, dCTP, dGTP, and dTTP) were treated at high temperatures and analyzed to determine residual amounts relative to those after incubation at 30°C. Most nucleotides were instable at 60°C (residual ratio: dATP, 68%; dCTP, 70%; dGTP, 71%; and dTTP, >99%). All of the nucleotides were clearly degraded into other forms when incubated at 80°C (dATP, 10%; dCTP, 26%; dGTP, 12%; and dTTP, 15%) and were completely degraded at 90°C (residual ratio, <0.2%). This suggests that the deoxyribonucleoside triphosphates are physicochemically unstable in the thermophiles.

3.5. Archaeal thermophiles: Smaller genomes

Genomic data were analyzed to compare the genome sizes of thermophiles (capable of growing at > 55°C) and mesophiles (capable of growing at 20–55°C). The genomes of thermophilic bacteria *Geobacillus* spp. (3.4 ± 0.3 Mb; n = 57) were smaller than those of phylogenetically related mesophiles, e.g., *B. subtilis* (4.1 ± 0.3 Mb; n = 100). The results were similar for archaeal methanogens, in which thermophiles had smaller genomes (1.7 ± 0.6 Mb; n = 20) than mesophiles (2.6 ± 0.8 Mb; n = 57). Archaeal thermophiles, such as *Pyrobaculum* (2.2 ± 1.6 Mb; n = 4), *Pyrococcus* (1.8 ± 0.1 Mb; n = 5), *Sulfolobus* (2.5 ± 0.2 Mb; n = 5), and *Thermococcus* (2.0 ± 0.1 Mb; n = 18) members, have much smaller genomes compared with archaeal mesophiles, such as *Haloarcula* (3.6 ± 1.2 Mb; n = 9), *Halococcus* (3.6 ± 0.4 Mb; n = 7), *Haloferax* (3.7 ± 0.4 Mb; n = 6), and *Halorubrum* (3.1 ± 0.8 Mb; n = 13) members. These data suggest that the thermophiles, especially archaeal thermophiles, tend to have smaller genomes than mesophiles.

	MK244	MK633
Transformation efficiency (per 10^6 recipients)		
E. coli BR397 donor	<1	300 ± 75
E. coli BR398 donor	55 ± 17	22 ± 3
E. coli BR408 donor	87 ± 14	34 ± 14
Mutation frequency (per 10^6 cells)		
Rifampicin resistance	12 ± 2	42 ± 8
Streptomycin resistance	7 ± 4	7 ± 2
Doubling time in LB medium (min)		
50°C	47 ± 6	42 ± 2
60°C	23 ± 2	21 ± 3
70°C	38 ± 7	32 ± 5
Doubling time in MM medium (min)		
50°C	100 ± 9	130 ± 20
60°C	83 ± 6	89 ± 2
70°C	ND	ND
pUCG18T retention rate (%)		
50°C	6 ± 3	58 ± 7
60°C	6 ± 4	79 ± 9
70°C	1 ± 1	64 ± 2
Cell yield (g wet weight per 20 ml culture)		
50°C	0.41 ± 0.01	0.41 ± 0.01
60°C	0.30 ± 0.03	0.36 ± 0.01
70°C	0.38 ± 0.03	0.41 ± 0.01

Table 3. Microbial properties of *G. kaustophilus* MK244 and MK633. Analyses were repeated more than three times. Data represent the mean ± standard error. ND, growth was not observed within 2 days.

3.6. Distribution of plasmids in archaeal thermophiles

Data mining showed that many thermophiles harbored plasmids, although not the majority. In *Archaea*, plasmids were identified frequently in *Sulfolobus* spp. (14 strains) and *Thermococcus* spp. (11 strains): pARN3 (26.2 kb), pARN4 (26.5 kb), pHEN7 (7.8 kb), pHVE14 (35.4 kb), pING1 (24.6 kb), pKEF9 (28.9 kb), pLD8501 (26.6 kb), pRN1 (5.4 kb), pRN2 (7.0 kb), pSOG1 (29.0 kb), pSOG2 (26.0 kb), pSSVx (5.7 kb), pXZ1 (7.0 kb), and pYN01 (42.2 kb) in *Sulfolobus islandicus;* pIT3 (5.0 kb), pMGB1 (28.0 kb), and pSSVi (5.7 kb) in *Sulfolobus solfataricus;* pTBMP1 (54.2 kb) in *Thermococcus barophilus;* an unnamed plasmid (3.6 kb) in *Thermococcus eurythermalis;* pTN1 (3.6 kb), pTN2 (13.0 kb), and pTN3 (18.3 kb) in *Thermococcus nautili;* an unnamed plasmid

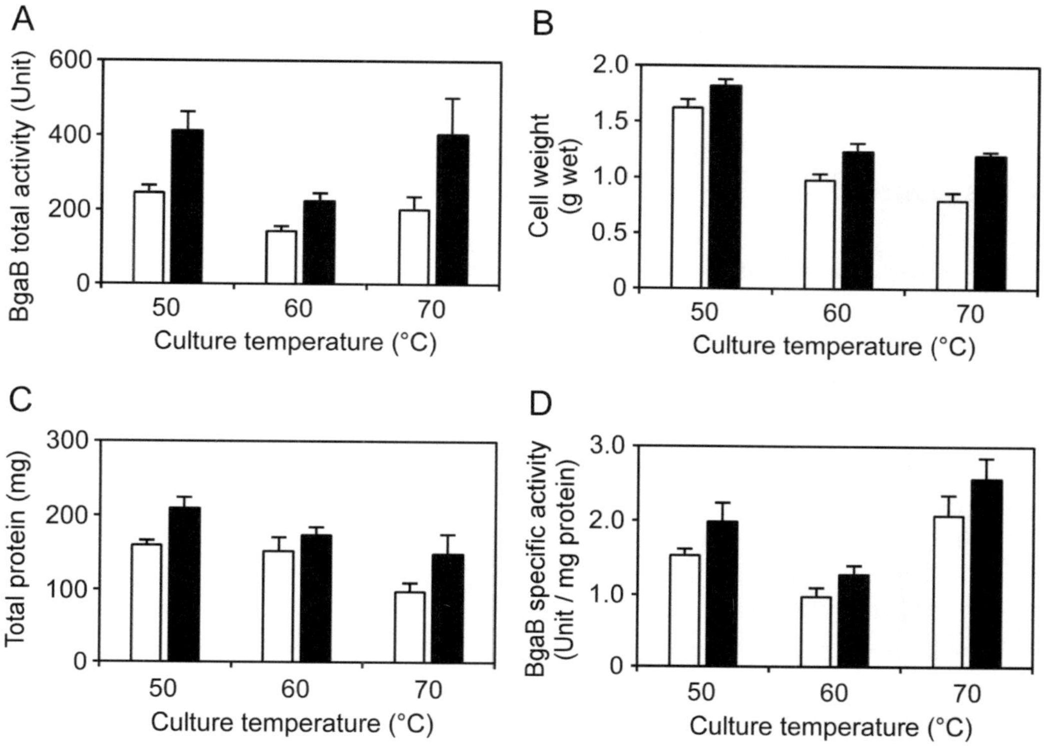

Figure 3. BgaB production by *G. kaustophilus* MK244$_{bgaB}$ and MK633$_{bgaB}$. These strains were cultured at 50, 60, and 70°C in medium (100 ml) and analyzed to determine the total activity in terms of intracellular BgaB (A), cell weight (B), intracellular total protein (C), and BgaB-specific activity (D). Data are expressed as the mean ± standard error (n = 4–5).

(49.1 kb) in *Thermococcus peptonophilus;* and pAMT7 (8.6 kb), pAMT11 (20.5 kb), pCIR10 (13.3 kb), pEXT9a (10.6 kb), pIRI33 (11.0 kb), pIRI48 (13.0 kb), and pT26-2 (21.6 kb) in *Thermococcus* spp. The other plasmids identified in archaeal thermophiles are as follows: pDSM2661_1 (58.4 kb) and pDSM2661_2 (16.6 kb) in *Methanocaldococcus jannaschii;* pMTBMA4 (4.4 kb) in *Methanothermobacter marburgensis;* pFV1 (13.5 kb), pFZ1 (11.0 kb), pME2001 (4.4 kb), and pME2200 (6.2 kb) in *Methanothermobacter thermautotrophicus;* pMETOK01 (14.9 kb) in *Methanothermococcus okinawensis;* pGT5 (3.4 kb) in *Pyrococcus abyssi;* and pTA1 (15.7 kb) in *Thermoplasma acidophilum.* In addition, several cryptic plasmids have been identified in archaeal thermophiles [28].

Plasmids are also distributed in bacterial thermophiles. In *Geobacillus* spp., seven strains of *Geobacillus* spp. harbored plasmids: pGS18 (plasmid length, 62.8 kb), pSTK1 (1.9 kb), pTB19 (11.9 kb), and an unnamed plasmid (21.7 kb) in *Geobacillus stearothermophilus;* pLW1071 (57.7 kb) in *Geobacillus thermodenitrificans;* pLDW-1 (48.7 kb) in *Geobacillus thermoleovorans;* and pBt40 (39.7 kb) in *Geobacillus* sp. In *Thermus* spp., 12 strains were identified as plasmid carriers. Their plasmids include pTA14 (14.4 kb), pTA16 (16.6 kb), pTA69 (69.9 kb), and pTA78 (78.7 kb) in *Thermus aquaticus;* pTB1 (342.8 kb) and pTB2 (10.3 kb) in *Thermus brockianus;* pTHEOS01 (271.7 kb) and pTHEOS02 (57.2 kb) in *Thermus oshimai;* pTP143 (143.3 kb) in *Thermus parvatiensis;* pTSC8 (8.4 kb) in *Thermus scotoductus;* and pTF62 (10.4 kb), pTHTHE1601 (440.0 kb), pTT8

(9.3 kb), pTT27 (232.6 kb), pTTJL1801 (265.9 kb), pTTJL1802 (142.7 kb), and pVV8 (81.2 kb) in *Thermus thermophilus*. In *Parageobacillus thermoglucosidans*, pGEOTH01 (80.8 kb), pGEOTH02 (19.6 kb), pNCI001 (83.9 kb), and pNCI002 (47.9 kb) were identified.

4. Discussion

In this study, we analyzed the effects of plasmid curing on thermophiles by characterizing *G. kaustophilus* MK244 and MK633 (**Table 3** and **Figure 3**). Both strains exhibited comparable growth at 50–70°C in LB and MM; therefore, pHTA426 had no positive effects on cell growth under standard conditions. The mutation frequencies were largely comparable between strains MK244 and MK633, although *G. kaustophilus* MK633 lacked the *gkp08* gene responsible for *dam*-like methylation (5′-GG^{6m}ATC-3′and 5′-G^{6m}ATCC-3′) and the *dam* methylation (5′-G^{6m}ATC-3′) is essential for DNA mismatch repair in *E. coli* [29]. In *B. subtilis* 168, DNA mismatch repair only involves *mutS* and *mutL* products, which do not depend on DNA methylation [30, 31], thereby suggesting that *G. kaustophilus* may use a mismatch repair system similar to the *B. subtilis* system rather than the *E. coli* system. In fact, the *G. kaustophilus* genome [17] contains *mutS* and *mutL* but not *mutH*, as found in *B. subtilis* 168.

A restriction-modification system generally protects the host microbe from transformation with exogenous DNA because the system cuts exogenous DNA that is not methylated by methyltransferase. However, a microbe can accept exogenous DNA that imitates the methylation pattern because a restriction-modification system is unable to cut this exogenous DNA [32]. In a previous study [12], we constructed *E. coli* strains BR397, BR398, and BR408 for conjugative plasmid transfer into *G. kaustophilus* HTA426. *E. coli* BR408 produces DNA that imitates the methylation pattern in *G. kaustophilus* HTA426. *E. coli* BR398 produces DNA with *dam* methylation, whereas *E. coli* BR397 produces methyl-free DNA. Although *G. kaustophilus* MK244 could not accept the pUCG18T plasmid transferred from the *dam*$^-$ strain *E. coli* BR397, *G. kaustophilus* MK633 accepted pUCG18T from *E. coli* BR397 as well as strains BR398 and BR408. These results can be explained by the elimination of *gkp09* from strain MK633 because the *gkp09* product digests methyl-free DNA but not DNA with *dam* methylation (5′-G^{6m}ATC-3′, which covers *gkp08* methylation (5′-GG^{6m}ATC-3′ and 5′-G^{6m}ATCC-3′. In addition, *G. kaustophilus* MK633 maintained pUCG18T with higher stability than strain MK244. This observation is also attributable to the elimination of *gkp09* because the *gkp09* product can occasionally digest endogenous plasmids that have not undergone *gkp08* methylation immediately after plasmid replication. This hypothesis is supported by the fact that *G. kaustophilus* MK244′ maintained pUCG18T as stably as strain MK633. Thus, *G. kaustophilus* MK633 acquired advantages compared with strain MK244 in terms of plasmid transformation and plasmid stability due to the elimination of a restriction-modification system along with pHTA426 curing.

An intriguing observation was that *G. kaustophilus* MK633 had a higher cell density in the stationary phase. In contrast to the advantages in terms of plasmid transformation and plasmid stability, this observation cannot be explained by the elimination of *gkp09* because *G. kaustophilus* MK244′ grew less efficiently than strain MK633. It was also interesting that strain MK633$_{bgaB}$ produced higher amounts of BgaB than MK244$_{bgaB}$ (**Figure 3A**). This observation is

http://dx.doi.org/10.5772/intechopen.70041

attributable mainly to the higher cell density of MK633$_{bgaB}$ (**Figure 3B**), as observed with strain MK633, and thus the higher protein yields from strain MK633$_{bgaB}$ (**Figure 3C**). In addition, this observation can be attributed to the higher BgaB productivity per cell because strain MK633$_{bgaB}$ had a higher BgaB specific activity (**Figure 3D**). Thus, these results suggest that the elimination of pHTA426 improved the cell density per culture and BgaB productivity per cell, thereby remarkably enhancing the production of BgaB.

Sodium dodecyl sulfate-polyacrylamide gel electrophoresis analysis showed that the crude extracts from *G. kaustophilus* MK244 and MK633 had negligible differences in terms of their protein compositions (data not shown). Therefore, it is unlikely that *G. kaustophilus* MK633 lost a nonessential protein that was abundantly synthesized from pHTA426, thereby reducing the energy burden to enhance the cell yield and BgaB productivity. Instead, these enhancements may be attributable to the reduced energy burden for plasmid replication. In fact, evidence suggests that plasmid maintenance places burdens on cell growth and/or metabolism [33–36]. Given that pHTA426 replicates as a single copy, this plasmid accounts for only 1.3% of total DNA; however, deoxyribonucleoside triphosphates are more unstable at higher temperatures, thereby suggesting that plasmid replication may place a considerable energy burden on thermophiles even though the plasmid is not extremely large or present in high copy numbers. This hypothesis is consistent with our genome data analysis, which showed that thermophiles have relatively smaller genomes than mesophiles, and the negative correlation between genome size and growth temperature reported by Sabath *et al* [37]. Overall, we consider that the lower energy burden incurred for DNA replication can explain why pHTA426 curing improved the cell density per culture and BgaB productivity per cell.

In conclusion, we demonstrated that pHTA426 curing was effective for improving the performance of a moderate thermophile, *G. kaustophilus* MK244. The cell density and protein productivity were presumably improved by the reduced amounts of energy required for DNA replication at high temperatures, so plasmid curing may be a simple approach for improving thermophiles in terms of these properties. In particular, this approach may be effective for archaeal thermophiles because they grow at extremely high temperatures and thus could have a greater energy burden on plasmid replication. Moreover, in archaeal thermophiles, plasmids may account for larger fractions of chromosomes than in moderate thermophiles because archaeal thermophile genomes are generally smaller. Therefore, plasmid curing could remarkably reduce the energy burden in archaeal thermophiles. We note that many archaeal thermophiles harbor plasmids, such as *S. solfataricus* P2 (carrying pSSVi) and *T. barophilus* MP (carrying pTBMP1), which have been studied as model acidophilic hyperthermophiles [38] and piezophilic hyperthermophiles [39], respectively. Even if these thermophiles harbor a single copy plasmid, our results suggest that plasmid curing can improve their performance in terms of the cell density and protein productivity.

Acknowledgements

The authors thank Dr. Hisashi Yagi of Tottori University for useful discussions. This study was supported by JSPS KAKENHI (Grant number 25450105).

Author details

Tatsuki Mizuno, Takashi Ohshiro and Hirokazu Suzuki*

*Address all correspondence to: hirokap@xpost.plala.or.jp

Department of Chemistry and Biotechnology, Graduate School of Engineering, Tottori University, Japan

References

[1] Wiegel J, Ljungdahl LG. The importance of thermophilic bacteria in biotechnology. Critical Reviews in Biotechnology. 1986;**3**:39-108

[2] Cripps RE, Eley K, Leak DJ, Rudd B, Taylor M, Todd M, Boakes S, Martin S, Atkinson T. Metabolic engineering of *Geobacillus thermoglucosidasius* for high yield ethanol production. Metabolic Engineering. 2009;**11**:398-408

[3] Georgieva TI, Ahring BK. Evaluation of continuous ethanol fermentation of dilute-acid corn stover hydrolysate using thermophilic anaerobic bacterium *Thermoanaerobacter* BG1L1. Applied Microbiology and Biotechnology. 2007;**77**:61-68

[4] Lin PP, Rabe KS, Takasumi JL, Kadisch M, Arnold FH, Liao JC. Isobutanol production at elevated temperatures in thermophilic *Geobacillus thermoglucosidasius*. Metabolic Engineering. 2014;**24**:1-8

[5] Shaw AJ, Podkaminer KK, Desai SG, Bardsley JS, Rogers SR, Thorne PG, Hogsett DA, Lynd LR. Metabolic engineering of a thermophilic bacterium to produce ethanol at high yield. Proceedings of the National Academy of Sciences of the United States of America. 2008;**105**:13769-13774

[6] Taylor MP, Eley KL, Martin S, Tuffin MI, Burton SG, Cowan DA. Thermophilic ethanologenesis: Future prospects for second-generation bioethanol production. Trends in Biotechnology. 2009;**27**:398-405

[7] Kanai T, Simons J-R, Tsukamoto R, Nakajima A, Omori Y, Matsuoka R, Beppu H, Imanaka T, Atomi H. Overproduction of the membrane-bound [NiFe]-hydrogenase in *Thermococcus kodakarensis* and its effect on hydrogen production. Frontiers in Microbiology. 2015;**6**:847

[8] Takami H, Inoue A, Fuji F, Horikoshi K. Microbial flora in the deepest sea mud of the Mariana Trench. FEMS Microbiology Letters. 1997;**152**:279-285

[9] Takami H, Nishi S, Lu J, Shinamura S, Takaki Y. Genomic characterization of thermophilic *Geobacillus* species isolated from the deepest sea mud of the Mariana Trench. Extremophiles. 2004;**8**:351-356

[10] Kobayashi J, Furukawa M, Ohshiro T, Suzuki H. Thermoadaptation-directed evolution of chloramphenicol acetyltransferase in an error-prone thermophile using improved procedures. Applied Microbiology and Biotechnology. 2015;**99**:5563-5572

[11] Kobayashi J, Tanabiki M, Doi S, Kondo A, Ohshiro T, Suzuki H. Unique plasmids generated via pUC replicon mutagenesis in an error-prone thermophile derived from *Geobacillus kaustophilus* HTA426. Applied and Environmental Microbiology. 2015;**81**:7625-7632

[12] Suzuki H, Yoshida K. Genetic transformation of *Geobacillus kaustophilus* HTA426 by conjugative transfer of host-mimicking plasmids. Journal of Microbiology and Biotechnology. 2012;**22**:1279-1287

[13] Suzuki H, Murakami A, Yoshida K. Counterselection system for *Geobacillus kaustophilus* HTA426 through disruption of *pyrF* and *pyrR*. Applied and Environmental Microbiology. 2012;**78**:7376-7383

[14] Suzuki H, Wada K, Furukawa M, Doi K, Ohshima T. A ternary conjugation system for the construction of DNA libraries for *Geobacillus kaustophilus* HTA426. Bioscience, Biotechnology, and Biochemistry. 2013;**77**:2316-2318

[15] Suzuki H, Yoshida K, Ohshima T. Polysaccharide-degrading thermophiles generated by heterologous gene expression in *Geobacillus kaustophilus* HTA426. Applied and Environmental Microbiology. 2013;**79**:5151-5158

[16] Wada K, Kobayashi J, Furukawa M, Doi K, Ohshiro T, Suzuki H. A thiostrepton resistance gene and its mutants serve as selectable markers in *Geobacillus kaustophilus* HTA426. Bioscience, Biotechnology, and Biochemistry. 2016;**80**:368-375

[17] Takami H, Takaki Y, Chee G-J, Nishi S, Shimamura S, Suzuki H, Matsui S, Uchiyama I. Thermoadaptation trait revealed by the genome sequence of thermophilic *Geobacillus kaustophilus*. Nucleic Acids Research. 2004;**32**:6292-6303

[18] Zheng C, He J, Wang Y, Wang M, Huang Z. Hydrocarbon degradation and bioemulsifier production by thermophilic *Geobacillus pallidus* strains. Bioresource Technology. 2011;**102**:9155-9161

[19] Kato T, Haruki M, Imanaka T, Morikawa M, Kanaya S. Isolation and characterization of long-chain-alkane degrading *Bacillus thermoleovorans* from deep subterranean petroleum reservoirs. Journal of Bioscience and Bioengineering. 2001;**91**:64-70

[20] Marchant R, Sharkey FH, Banat IM, Rahman TJ, Perfumo A. The degradation of *n*-hexadecane in soil by thermophilic geobacilli. FEMS Microbiology Ecology. 2006;**56**:44-54

[21] Wang L, Tang Y, Wang S, Liu R, Liu M, Zhang Y, Liang F, Feng L. Isolation and characterization of a novel thermophilic *Bacillus* strain degrading long-chain *n*-alkanes. Extremophiles. 2006;**10**:347-356

[22] Shimura M, Mukerjee-Dhar G, Kimbara K, Nagato H, Kiyohara H, Hatta T. Isolation and characterization of a thermophilic *Bacillus* sp. JF8 capable of degrading polychlorinated biphenyls and naphthalene. FEMS Microbiology Letters. 1999;**178**:87-93

[23] Sood N, Lal B. Isolation and characterization of a potential paraffin-wax degrading thermophilic bacterial strain *Geobacillus kaustophilus* TERI NSM for application in oil wells with paraffin deposition problems. Chemosphere. 2008;**70**:1445-1451

[24] Tomita K, Ikeda N, Ueno A. Isolation and characterization of a thermophilic bacterium, *Geobacillus thermocatenulatus*, degrading nylon 12 and nylon 66. Biotechnology Letters. 2003;**25**:1743-1746

[25] Amartey SA, Leak DJ, Hartley BS. Development and optimization of a defined medium for aerobic growth of *Bacillus stearothermophilus* LLD-15. Biotechnology Letters. 1991;**13**:621-626

[26] Suzuki H, Kobayashi J, Wada K, Furukawa M, Doi K. Thermoadaptation-directed enzyme evolution in an error-prone thermophile derived from *Geobacillus kaustophilus* HTA426. Applied and Environmental Microbiology. 2015;**81**:149-158

[27] Naito N, Kusano K, Kobayashi I. Selfish behavior of restriction–modification systems. Science. 1995;**267**:897-899

[28] Zillig W, Prangishvilli D, Schleper C, Elferink M, Holz I, Albers S, Janekovic D, Götz D. Viruses, plasmids and other genetic elements of thermophilic and hyperthermophilic *Archaea*. FEMS Microbiology Reviews. 1996;**18**:225-236

[29] Kunkel TA, Erie DA. DNA mismatch repair. Annual Review of Biochemistry. 2005;**74**:681-710

[30] Pillon MC, Lorenowicz JJ, Uckelmann M, Klocko AD, Mitchell RR, Chung YS, Modrich P, Walker GC, Simmons LA, Friedhoff P, Guarné A. Structure of the endonuclease domain of MutL: Unlicensed to cut. Molecular Cell. 2010;**39**:145-151

[31] Simmons LA, Davies BW, Grossman AD, Walker GC. β clamp directs localization of mismatch repair in *Bacillus subtilis*. Molecular Cell. 2008;**29**:291-301

[32] Suzuki H. Host-mimicking strategies in DNA methylation for improved bacterial transformation. In: Dricu A, editor. Methylation—From DNA, RNA and Histones to Diseases and Treatment. Rijeka: InTech; 2012. pp. 219-236

[33] Helling RB, Kinney T, Adams J. The maintenance of plasmid-containing organisms in populations of *Escherichia coli.* Journal of General Microbiology. 1981;**123**:129-141

[34] Jones KL, Kim SW, Keasling JD. Low-copy plasmids can perform as well as or better than high-copy plasmids for metabolic engineering of bacteria. Metabolic Engineering. 2000;**2**:328-338

[35] Ow DS, Nissom PM, Philip R, Oh SK, Yap MG. Global transcriptional analysis of metabolic burden due to plasmid maintenance in *Escherichia coli* DH5α during batch fermentation. Enzyme and Microbial Technology. 2006;**39**:391-398

[36] Seo J, Balley JE. Effects of recombinant plasmid content on growth properties and cloned gene product formation in *Escherichia coli*. Biotechnology & Bioengineering. 1985;**27**:1668-1674

[37] Sabath N, Ferrada E, Barve A, Wagner A. Growth temperature and genome size in bacteria are negatively correlated, suggesting genomic streamlining during thermal adaptation. Genome Biology and Evolution. 2013;**5**:966-977

[38] Berkner S, Lipps G. Genetic tools for *Sulfolobus* spp.: Vectors and first applications. Archives of Microbiology. 2008;**190**:217-230

[39] Thiel A, Michoud G, Moalic Y, Flament D, Jebbar M. Genetic manipulations of the hyperthermophilic piezophilic archaeon *Thermococcus barophilus*. Applied and Environmental Microbiology. 2014;**80**:2299-2306